getfitnow

THE HIGH SCHOOL
ATHLETE
BASEBALL

THE COMPLETE PROGRAM FOR STRENGTH AND CONDITIONING
★ FOR PLAYERS AND COACHES ★

MIKE VOLKMAR   FOREWORD BY JOSH BELL

Hatherleigh Press is committed to preserving and protecting the natural resources of the earth. Environmentally responsible and sustainable practices are embraced within the company's mission statement.

Visit us at www.hatherleighpress.com.

THE HIGH SCHOOL ATHLETE: BASEBALL

Library of Congress Cataloging-in-Publication Data is available upon request.
ISBN: 978-1-57826-822-1

All Hatherleigh Press titles are available for bulk purchase, special promotions, and premiums. For information about reselling and special purchase opportunities, please call 1-800-528-2550 and ask for the Special Sales Manager.

Cover and Interior Design by Carolyn Kasper

10 9 8 7 6 5 4 3 2 1
Printed in the United States

CONTENTS

FOREWORD
by Josh Bell, MLB All-Star

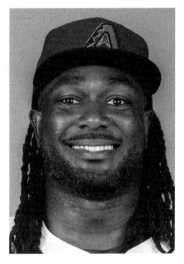

Though I'm fortunate enough to be a professional baseball player today, my athletic journey started at a young age. My father laid down a pretty strict regimen for me to follow in regard to my physicality and athletic performance; from ages 4–16, I played no less than two sports a year. Basketball was my favorite, as it happens, followed by baseball (which I was obviously best at), but I also dabbled in soccer and track and field. My father made sure I spent hours each week shooting, dribbling, hitting off of a pitching machine, throwing at targets; he also created different workouts for me to do before and after specific sport training. For example, walking lunges while loaded down with a weight vest and jogging backwards were two workouts that I did following each of my baseball practices in high school, a half-mile of each. In this way, my dad instilled in me the idea that, so long as I was out-working all of my competitors, I could continue to succeed on the field and on the court.

Since my junior year of high school, I've focused solely on baseball. (At the time, this was to ensure I kept my athletic scholarship to play at the University of Texas.) I've been competing at a high level and holding my own against my peers, for which I had my athleticism and work ethic to thank. All in all, I'm a firm believer in outworking the competition. My father made sure I was always working uncomfortably hard; throughout my journey, this trait has always been my strength in every sport I've ever played.

If I could give my younger self some advice, I'd tell him to focus much more on the dietary and recovery side of health. Like most kids, I felt like I could eat whatever I wanted, with Gatorade being my drink of choice for many years. Knowing what I know now, I'd tell myself to cut out all refined sugar—NO sports drinks, NO desserts, NO ice cream. I'd also tell myself to stay away from fatty or starchy foods—NO fast food, NO processed meats. I'd also recommend he cultivate a stronger focus on recovery, so that neither my nutrition nor my sleep routine would get in the way of my performance.

Our bodies are capable of doing so much more than we think, but proper care and foundational health impacts the height of our physical peak. As long as you're fueling your body to allow it to recover, the sky is the limit for your athletic ability.

— JOSH BELL, MLB All-Star

THE HIGH SCHOOL ATHLETE METHOD

This book is more than just 100 baseball-specific killer workouts. This book is a compilation of workouts, based on an age-appropriate and holistic development model of **motivation, nutrition** and **training**, based on multiple methodologies of athlete development. It is intended for use by baseball coaches, baseball players, parents of baseball players, and strength and conditioning coaches at or nearing the high school level. I truly believe the foundations of this book mimic the most successful college baseball programs.

MOTIVATION

The current generation of players is different from the ones who played 20 years ago. This book explores the mindset of a successful player in the modern game of baseball. While some kids still need "a kick in the pants," others are motivated by ego or held back by fear. How do you know what motivates each of your players? How do you deal with different personalities?

Motivation no longer consists of blindly yelling at your players or making them run laps or poles for discipline. Instead, we will be examining the different development stages that players go through to further our understanding of how to motivate them effectively.

Remember, the best training program in the world means nothing if you can't get players to "buy in."

NUTRITION

Nutrition is the newest frontier in high school level athletics. **Athletes eat and train—they do not diet and exercise.** Sports nutrition has officially made its way down from the professional and collegiate ranks, and high school athletes are learning the importance of nutrition. However, they are getting overwhelmed in the process.

Without a qualified coach to teach proper nutrition and sort through the barrage of information provided by unfiltered internet searches about fad diets and supplements, kids are more confused than ever. This book provides a simplified "food first" approach that can help all players. We have also provided a list of online resources to help provide access to easy-to-understand information; see the Resources section at the end.

TRAINING

Coaches, this book aims to build up your freshman and sophomore players by focusing on exercises that put them into a position of success. **Training can be so much more than an endless repetition of squats, benches, and plyometrics.** Using a "slow burn," 4-year training plan, this book programs specifically for each season, with progressions and advancements for every player.

Players, I know all you care about is running faster, throwing 90, or hitting bombs. Rest assured—every workout in this book brings you closer to those goals! Don't believe me? Take it from MiLB Strength and Conditioning Coach for the Philadelphia Phillies, Bruce Peditto: "In my time working as a strength and conditioning coach in professional baseball, I have come across athletes with a wide variety of training backgrounds. From high school to college draft picks to young international players, there is one thing that seems to hold consistent—the athletes with the better training background seem to advance more quickly through the levels. The better control a player has over his body, the more strength, the more speed, the more likely he is to stand out amongst his peers. If you look at the perennial all-stars at the major league level, their work ethics are beyond those of the average player and most of their training regimens are comprised of the same elements that are covered here in this book."

PART I: MOTIVATION

This section focuses on what we'll refer to as the "art" of strength and conditioning and is presented with both athletes and coaches in mind. The information provided applies equally to both aspects of baseball training—coaching technique and athletic performance—but athletes and coaches should approach the training with the mindset that best suits their respective positions.

COACHES

At the end of the day, coaching in its purest form is the art of recognizing and adapting to situations in order to optimize your athletes' performance—both on the field and in the weight room. The best coaches are those who can adapt and customize their programming to fit the specific needs of the individual athlete (injury history, emotional and physical needs, level of commitment, etc.), rather than sticking to one set program that every athlete must fit into (or bust). I believe coaches should write their programs in pencil, not pen, so to speak.

However, what about those aspects of training that don't directly relate to an athlete's physical condition on any given day? An athlete's motivation, their drive to push themselves and succeed, to live up to your expectations, is directly related to their mental, emotional, social, and cognitive development—and how a coach navigates those factors during training directly determines how well an athlete will perform.

Generally speaking, people are experiencing a combination of human emotions at any given time. It is a coach's job to find out what makes them tick and push the right buttons at the right time. This allows you to gain their trust and increase their level of effort, which helps your training programs become more effective.

Being more mindful of the impact of each individual's personality types, attitudes, behaviors, and drives can help you to mold your coaching to the individual and their situation.

ATHLETES

What motivates you? Whether you have the drive not just to succeed, but to excel, is going to come down to keeping your internal and external motivations balanced and working in tandem to push you to new heights. Your love of the game (your internal motivation) should pair with your dreams of potential awards, scholarships or publicity (external motivations).

However, while striving for that "Player of the Year" distinction or headlines in the local paper are visceral, intense motivators, your pure enjoyment of the game and the sense of satisfaction felt from playing well should be paramount. So decide now whether you're willing to focus on the **process**—practices, time in the weight room, film study—rather than just the **outcome,** win or lose. As a player, you will find increased confidence in your abilities when you focus on the process and use external motivators as a bonus.

MOTIVATING PLAYERS

oaches: never forget that you're coaching people, not robots. You must understand and know your players in order to properly motivate them. You also need to have the flexibility to color outside the lines of your precisely prepared spreadsheet workouts. Therefore, you should be driven by principles, not rules.

This understanding begins with a proper knowledge of how exactly we take in and process new information.

THE FOUR STAGES OF LEARNING

When developing a program, you must always account for the four stages of learning that every human goes through.

Unconscious Incompetence

This is the starting point for everyone. At this stage (typically during freshman year), the athlete is taught the benefits and importance of the skills and/or exercises they will be learning. Prior to this point, they may not be aware of these skills/exercises, and may not even appreciate their own deficiencies in this area. Until this lack of awareness is overcome, no progress can be made.

Conscious Incompetence

This will typically take place during sophomore year. The athlete gains a level of appreciation for the skills and exercises they're being taught, usually by experiencing some failure on their way to progressing to competence.

Conscious Competence

This is where the bulk of your efforts should be directed. During junior year, the athlete can reliably perform the skills and exercises, but requires a great deal focus, concentration, and hard work in order to perform correctly. Without proper concentration and proper conditioning, the skill or exercise is still difficult or impossible for them to reliably perform.

Unconscious Competence

By this stage, the athlete has practiced enough and been put through enough situations using the skills and exercises being taught that using them has become second nature. There is little to no concentration required to perform the skill correctly. While some athletes never reach this point, this is an achievable target goal for senior year.

This is a somewhat simplistic and linear way of describing these four stages. It is intended only to illustrate the "slow burn" process you must go through as a coach during the early high school years.

COACHING PROGRESSION AND THE FOUR STAGES

Now that you've seen the four stages—which should seem familiar to you, if you have any prior experience coaching athletes—it's time to talk specifics. How do these stages apply to one's coaching philosophies? How do you program for these developmental categories?

1. Do not overwhelm your incoming freshman.

The weight room can be an intimidating place for incoming freshman. While modern athletes are beginning their training younger and younger, this does not prepare them for the intensity of a full team lift in the varsity weight room. Focus on communication, encouragement, and enrichment, and avoid putting them in situations where they are immediately called upon to perform above their level. Adam Feit, MS, CSCS*D, Coordinator of Physical and Mental Performance, Doctoral Candidate of Sport and Exercise Psychology at Springfield College, says, "Competence breeds confidence."

2. Do not overcoach your freshman and sophomores.

One of the biggest issues in Youth Sports Specialization is parent coaching—which can be at once overwhelming and inconsistent, teaching low self-confidence and bad habits. If combined with an overemphasis on winning at a young age, you'll find that your younger players cannot think for themselves. Therefore, choose exercises that are safe and create an environment for the athlete to learn.

For example, consider the deadlift. Do not allow a first- or second-year player (who you have yet to see lift and therefore cannot properly assess) to deadlift a heavy load from the floor with a straight barbell during their first workout. There are two reasons for this restriction: 1) it is obviously dangerous, but also 2) could crush their confidence by embarrassing a player in front of their peers or risking injury.

Remember, emotional security is a big part of learning in the early years of high school. Put your younger players in a position to succeed with a light barbell RDL or a Dumbbell Goblet Squat.

- The danger of the exercise is very low because the weight is lower and easy to grab.

- It creates emotional security because it can be performed away from the platforms if necessary.

- By having the athlete stand directly above the kettlebell, dumbbell or light barbell, it allows them the freedom to tinker with body positions and angles. This keeps the need for cues minimal and allows for encouragement on what they are doing correctly.

Positive progressions like this (as opposed to asking your players to do something they are not ready to do) provide the building blocks for building a relationship with your players. This even applies to the advanced younger athlete, or those who are very persistent that they are ready for the barbell. As a coach, I do not believe in holding any one athlete back, but I still use prudence when making exceptions. If you have a freshman or new sophomore who has clearly spent time in the weight room, allow them to go through the simple progressions quickly to prove to you and themselves that they are truly ready for the barbell.

SELF-DISCOVERY

The principle of self-discovery—what some call a "light bulb" moment—is incredibly important to the growth of an athlete. An athlete who is allowed to learn from failure (safely, of course) will learn lifelong lessons in the weight room about themselves, their strengths, and their limitations. Guided discovery and experimental learning are critical elements in the discussion of motor learning behavior.

For example, let's say your 6'3" sophomore right fielder has his heart set on the Barbell Back Squat. He wants to emulate his role model, the 5'9" senior center fielder, a future college player who is crushing squats with three plates on each side of the bar. However, the long, weak levers of the sophomore athlete do not allow the sophomore to back squat with that amount of weight; when he does attempt heavy weights, his knees hurt the day after.

As a coach, you see this situation and let your sophomore know that the Front Squat or Goblet Squat would allow him to reach better depth and provide less stress on his knees. But as his coach, you can see the intensity in his eyes when he talks about the back squat, so you give him some encouragement but caution him that his knees will continue to hurt going down this path.

A few weeks later, he approaches you during warm-up and says his knees are still sore and the weight on the back squat is stuck; maybe it *is* time for a change, he says. As the coach, I would praise his maturity in accepting change, while also telling him to take a few days off from squats to allow his knees to rest. Once he's feeling great again, you can tackle the Dumbbell Goblet Squat and work on building him up to the Barbell Front Squat. To seal the deal, a few days later, during his first squat session back, you ask the senior whom he admires to go over and give the underclassman a few words of encouragement about trusting the process.

I see some version of these events every year in my high school gym. Some kids learn best by learning from their own mistakes. You, as the coach, must have the patience to allow that to happen. As Coach Brett Bartholomew once said, "The job is to prepare the athlete for the path, not the path for the athlete."

3. Remember that you are coaching visual learners.

Today's players grow up online, taught by YouTube videos and TikToks. Demonstrating the exercise for them yourself, or else having them watch a video of proper technique, is very beneficial—especially in the early stages.

Keep your verbal cues to a minimum and allow your athletes the freedom to learn by watching and imitating.

4. Stay positive (most of the time).

Famed basketball coach Phil Jackson once described the best ratio of "specific, truthful, positive praise" to "specific, constructive criticism" that coaches should use with their players. Jackson said the ideal ratio is 5:1 (five positives to each correction), though he admits that his ratio with his players was closer to 3:1.

Jackson added, "Players often hear only the corrections and can become frustrated or angry at themselves and their coaches. It is a constant battle for coaches to stay positive and find new ways to get their players to hear and accept the positives so that they stay open to the occasional need for correction."

Put simply: if you are constantly yelling at your players, your voice becomes dull to their ears—they start tuning you out. Get your players' attention by raising your voice only at opportune times for greater effect.

5. Allow peer-to-peer mentorship and coaching.

I also call this one "positive peer pressure." Allow your four-year seniors to coach and mentor your freshman and new sophomores. If you've taught and coached your seniors correctly, their advice should be an extension of your method when teaching the fundamentals to the younger athletes. Positive peer-to-peer interactions can be very powerful. Think back to your time in high school. Did a senior whom you revered ever reach out and help you? If they did, you probably still remember that interaction. Your athletes can have those moments as well, if you allow them.

BIPOLAR COACHING

The term "bipolar coaching" comes from strength coach Joe DeFranco in an interview he did in 2013. I define bipolar coaching as using gender-specific language to accomplish specific goals. In other words, I coach boys differently from girls—because boys and girls respond differently to certain methods.

With boys, you'll hear me use words like jacked," "huge," and "big." "Shoulder presses are going to get you jacked and help you fill out that uniform!" I'll say. Or maybe, "Squat are going to get you huge so you can dominate in the base paths!"

For the girls, I use terms like "strong, "lean," and "powerful." When prescribing the same exercises (with similar goals), it might sound like this: "Shoulder presses are going make you look leaner, especially for prom season!" or, "Squats are going to get you stronger to help you go first to third faster!"

Same exercises, similar goals, but a different message.

Of course, regardless of how you communicate, athletes do not care how much you know until they know how much you care. Male or female, the trick is to find out what makes your athletes tick and push those buttons to get the best out of them.

(For a deeper dive into coaching female athletes from a male's perspective, check out Athletes Acceleration's *Complete Guide to Training the Female Athlete*. In there, they have a lesson called "Training The Other Side" in which Bobby Smith gives his experiences coaching all levels of female athletes. Another great resource on this topic is *Conscious Coaching: The Art and Science of Building Buy-In* by Brett Bartholomew. In his book, Brett breaks down the different personalities you may find in your weight room or on your team and gives tips on how to best connect with each type of personality.)

MENTAL TOUGHNESS

We all want our athletes mentally tougher. We all want our athlete to rebound from failure. How does a player respond after striking out for a third time in one game?

Adam Feit, Coordinator of Physical and Mental Performance at Springfield College, recently presented his "4Ps Framework" at a conference I attended while writing this book. After hearing him speak, I just had to include some of his highlights:

- **PREPARE** for the journey (practice, lift, game) ahead

- **PUSH** past their limits

- **PERSIST** through adversity and failure

- **PERFORM** with high character and fortitude

PREPARE

Preparation involves goal-setting, especially setting SMART goals that are specific, measurable, attainable, realistic, and time-bound (see my section on *Testing and Strength Ratios* on page 130). As coaches, keep things realistic; do not test your player's 1 mile run expecting faster than 60 second times. It also involves creating pre-performance routines. Focus on what is within your control: breathing, "facts not feelings," positive visualization, etc. Create short routines in the on-deck circle, between pitches, and between sets.

PUSH

Pushing involves reframing your thought process. Feit says "Reframe to reload"—in other words, turn a "but" into an "and." Maybe you (the athlete) are feeling overwhelmed about homework, a test on Friday, a late night training session. You start to make an excuse: "But I have a training session…" or you can turn that "but" into an "and." You get the privilege of going to school *and* training for the sport you love.

Feit also suggests that you "Segment the suck." This means to break down a large, imposing task into smaller, more manageable sections. This could be an attempt at a new 5-rep max on squats; instead of overwhelming yourself by thinking, "How on Earth am I going to squat this weight five times?" think, "All I have is 5 sets of 1 rep. I can squat this weight once."

PERSIST

Persistence involves controlling the controllable. Take control of *your* attitude, preparation, and effort. Ignore other peoples' feelings, opinions, actions, and mistakes. Feit says to focus on the *facts* and the *process*, not other's feelings and the product. He then goes one step further and asks athletes to "Concentrate to crush." Feit believes that mentally tough athletes can focus on four key areas: relevance, duration, awareness, and flexibility.

- Keep your focus only on the **relevant** details that affect your success.

- Maintain a high **duration** of concentration by taking one play at a time.

- Be **aware** of all the people trying to distract and steal from your attention.

- Be **flexible** in life, the weight room, and on the field. Life can change at any moment.

PERFORM

Performing involves managing your emotions. *Select* the situation that puts you in the best position to succeed. *Modify* a task (be it squats, deadlifts, or hitting a curve ball) to allow for success, not failure. *Deploy* your attention away from worrisome activities. *Change* your perspective on any situation to put yourself in control. *Respond* with positive actions (a healthy meal, a workout, or positive body language), not negative reactions (like diving into a pint of ice cream after a bad game, skipping a workout because you lack motivation, or showing your opponent you're tired). Finally, use music to psych you up and down. Play motivating music close to game time, not three hours before. Listen to calming music after your workout, during your cooldown, to help you reflect and to switch from athlete to student.

As coaches, techniques and methods of motivating your players have grown exponentially since we were players. It is imperative that we accept and grow in terms of mental conditioning and strength just as we grow and adapt our philosophies on the hit-and-run or bunting with a runner on second base. Likewise, as players, you have the responsibility to take control of your emotional state. Eliminate the noise in order to focus all your attention on becoming the best player you can become—that is your first responsibility.

TRAINING MODELS

The following training model gives a better look at the developmental phases players go through. Each model breaks down the physical and emotional traits of your athletes. Again, the better you understand your athletes, the better you can motivate them.

THE LONG-TERM ATHLETE DEVELOPMENT (LTAD)

Developed by the MLB and USA Baseball, the following model outlines the different phases we see in the growth of an athlete. (Visit usabltad. com for more information on all the stages, the aims of the program, development pathway stages, key principles, and key definitions.)

1. **Activate.** Until age 7. Kids are introduced to baseball through a style of play that promotes fun, play, and success.

2. **Discover.** From ages 7–12. Basic baseball skills are learned and developed in a positive environment.

3. **Progress.** From ages 12–14. Baseball skills continue to develop. Proper arm care planning begins. Players should still spend more time training than in competition.

4. **Develop.** From ages 14–16. Players may start picking a preferred position. Players may also choose to specialize in baseball, but multiple sport participation is encouraged.

5. **Apply.** From ages 16–18. Increased intensity in all facets from the Develop stage. (An advanced track is available for the Develop and Apply stages, aimed at those players projected to play in college or professionally.)

6. **Excel.** From age 19+. All phases of baseball development are maximized by expert coaches.

7. **Inspire.** Includes people of all ages involved in the game at any level or position, be it coach, player, or umpire.

"DEVELOP" AND "APPLY"

We focus on the Develop and Apply stages in this book. The Develop level refers to first- and second-year players, while the Apply phase refers to third- and fourth-year players on varsity teams.

Develop Level Key Points

- Focus is more on skill training and physical development and less on trying to win.

- Focus is on building the proper process vs. stressing the outcome.

- Players are allowed to fail safely.

- Provides space for a little fun and allows for socialization to avoid future burnout.

- Emphasis is on interpersonal skills, teamwork, and communication skills.

Apply Level Key Points

- Training intensity increases.

- Players can either choose to specialize in baseball or continue to play a second sport.

- High-volume and high-intensity training begins to occur year-round. Athletes also start to follow a more consistent, year-round training schedule.

- Greater emphasis on competition; players begin to participate in showcases and college camps.

THE NSCA TEN PILLARS FOR SUCCESSFUL LONG-TERM ATHLETIC DEVELOPMENT

1. Long-term athletic development pathways should accommodate for the highly individualized and non-linear nature of the growth and development of youth.

2. Youth of all ages, abilities and aspirations should engage in long-term athletic development programs that promote both physical fitness and psychosocial well-being.

3. All youth should be encouraged to enhance physical fitness from early childhood, with a primary focus on motor skill and muscular strength development.

4. Long-term athletic development pathways should encourage an early sampling approach for youth that promotes and enhances a broad range of motor skills.

5. Health and wellbeing of the child should always be the central tenet of long-term athletic development programs.

6. Youth should participate in physical conditioning that helps reduce the risk of injury to ensure their on-going participation in long-term athletic development programs.

7. Long-term athletic development programs should provide all youth with a range of training modes to enhance both health- and skill-related components of fitness.

8. Practitioners should use relevant monitoring and assessment tools as part of a long-term athletic development strategy.

9. Practitioners working with youth should systematically progress and individualize training programs for successful long-term athletic development.

10. Qualified professionals and sound pedagogical approaches are fundamental to the success of long-term athletic development programs.

POTENTIAL BENEFITS OF PLAYING MULTIPLE SPORTS

I asked my friend, professional baseball player, coach, and overall great human being, Jon Schwind, to write about his experience playing multiple sports growing up and how that affected his trajectory to professional sports.

Jon was a multi-sport athlete in high school and played college baseball at Marist College, where he was drafted by the Pittsburgh Pirates in 2011. He also spends the off-season coaching at the College at Brockport and coaching Challenger Baseball.

"I grew up in an athletic family with three older brothers who were always either outside playing in the neighborhood, or wreaking havoc inside, usually breaking something along the way. From my first memory, my childhood was consistently shaped around following their path. Whatever they did, I wanted to do better. Wherever they went, I wanted to get there faster. So naturally, I watched their every move, and that included watching them play sports.

"I wouldn't say that the sports I played growing up were really forced; more, copied. I thought that the sports our family played were soccer, hockey, and baseball. Other games were fun and enjoyable, but they were more reserved for the street or backyards of our neighborhood. I wasn't ever told that these were the organized sports I was going to play; it was more something I just assumed. Fall was for soccer, winter was for hockey, and summer was for baseball.

"Regardless of the choice, or lack thereof, that I had in what I played, I never solely focused on one sport for longer than its yearly season. Once one sport was over, it was time to start preparing for the next. This was most noticeable during the transition from the summer to the fall (baseball to soccer). Having not conditioned like a soccer player all summer, I would start running a week before soccer tryouts started and would expect to be ready. And somehow, after a few rusty days, my skill would catch up quickly and I would compete at a respectable level.

"Most people would say that I was able to do this because I was 'naturally gifted' or I was 'born athletic.' I couldn't disagree more. My athletic skills were no doubt developed by the variety of activities I did as an adolescent. I *never* specialized movement to a certain sport, and I for sure didn't train the entire year for one sport season. Rather, I did a little bit of everything. On a summer day, I might wake up and ride my bike to my friend's house about a mile away, play some pick-up basketball in his backyard, transition to some sort of street game involving a scooter and mini-soccer ball, ride our bikes back to my house, eat some lunch, play about 10 games of ping pong in my basement (until my mother would kick us out of the house or a paddle would get broken), ride our bikes back to my friend's house, go swimming in his pool, play a 2-on-2 football game, head back to my house for dinner, and play a baseball game that night. Most people might say a day this jam-packed is overwhelming, that kids don't have enough energy and we need to protect them from getting injured. What a limited perspective!

"The prevalence of playing multiple sports is decreasing in American society. In a time where video games are more popular than outdoor activities, youth sports are at an all-time low. Yes, we have our staple sports; however, so many children have never even picked up a tennis racket or hockey stick. Not only does this need to change to save sports in general, but it needs to change to help promote athleticism. Every sport has a wide variety of movements and skills that it repeats. They are all similar, yet all vastly different. By playing multiple sports, so many different skills—skills that are useful across the entire category of sports—are improved. All of this is necessary to create a much more complete athletic experience, one that can allow an athlete to reach their *full* potential.

"I wouldn't change one thing about my sports experience during my childhood. I developed talents and learned lessons from those days of riding my bike down the street. Specialization would've limited my ability to athletically improvise. I say, play sports, get athletic—and be curious!"

—*Jon Schwind, trainoffthegrid.com*

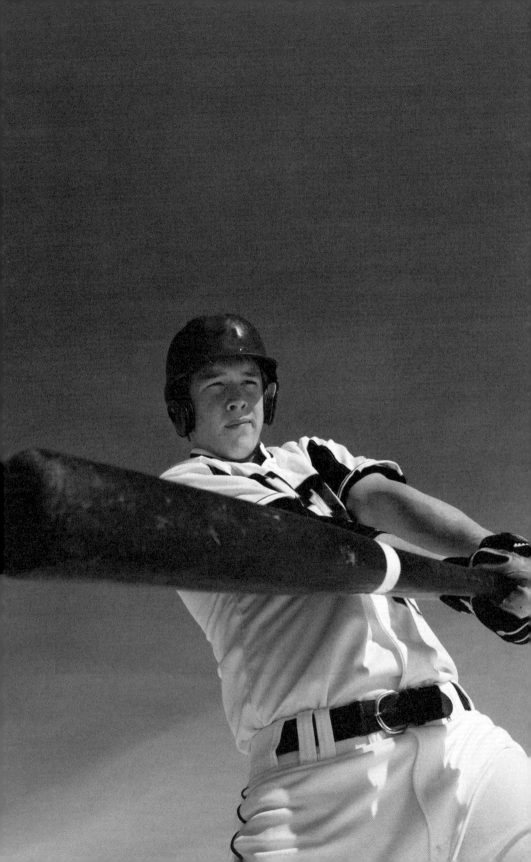

PART II: NUTRITION

Sports nutrition is the new frontier in improved sports performance at the high school level. The importance of sports nutrition as a field, and how impactful it can be on an athlete's recovery and physical development, has trickled down from the professional and collegiate level to apply to high school athletes. Proper nutrition is vital for any aspiring championship team and every single athlete involved. As Vince Lombardi once said, "The difference between a successful person and others is not a lack of strength, not a lack of knowledge, but rather a lack of will." In other words, a player who trains hard but does not eat like a champion is resigning himself to mediocrity, never quite reaching his full potential. A player who trains hard and does eat like a champion, however, sets himself up for success—because everything he does is working towards his goals.

An athlete's ability to recover and grow from their workouts is directly related to their nutritional intake. Nutrition also directly affects your ability to lose body fat and/or gain muscle. In this section, we'll be going over everything you need to know to set an athlete on the right nutritional track for victory and personal records.

Remember: no one has more control over an athlete's nutrition than the athlete themselves. There is very little you can be in complete control of, especially when playing a team sport, but taking your nutrition seriously is one of the biggest factors in the pursuit of athletic excellence—and it happens to be one of the few within your control.

NUTRITION BASICS FOR YOUNGER ATHLETES

On the field and off it, nutrition is key! For you to maximize your performance and recover quickly, you must eat right. Having consistent, good eating habits will bring your conditioning, speed and strength performances to the next level.

Choosing the correct foods in the right proportions and at the right times can make all the difference between success and defeat. A properly fueled and hydrated athlete is primed to perform at their best while minimizing the chances of fatigue, injury and dehydration.

Not only is nutrition both preparative and preventative, nutrition also provides the critical "trigger" for translating practice and weight training into increases in strength, power, speed and agility.

RELATIONSHIP BETWEEN TRAINING AND NUTRITION

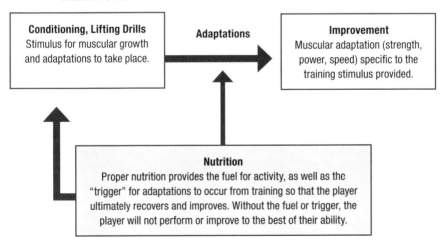

Conditioning, Lifting Drills
Stimulus for muscular growth and adaptations to take place.

Adaptations

Improvement
Muscular adaptation (strength, power, speed) specific to the training stimulus provided.

Nutrition
Proper nutrition provides the fuel for activity, as well as the "trigger" for adaptations to occur from training so that the player ultimately recovers and improves. Without the fuel or trigger, the player will not perform or improve to the best of their ability.

Simply put, lifting and conditioning serve as a stimulus to the body, and answering that stimulus with proper rest and nutrition is what allows for muscular adaptions in speed, strength, and power.

The following diagram illustrates what younger (high school) baseball players should really focus on in regard to nutrition. But walk into any high school weight room or locker room and you'll probably find that this chart is flipped on its head. Instead of kids discussing what they had for breakfast or what healthy choices they plan on making, they're talking about the latest "muscle building" supplement or "pre-workout" energy drink they picked up from the local store.

Comparing Magnitudes

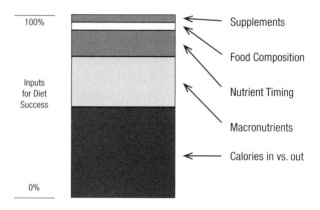

Be sure to teach your players about:

- **Calories in versus calories out:** Finding a balance of calories to achieve an ideal body composition.

- **Macronutrients:** Focusing on fruits, vegetables, lean proteins, healthy fats, and pre- and post-game carbohydrates.

- **Nutrient timing:** Stressing the importance of fueling up for a hard practice/game and refueling after a big lift or run to help recovery and performance.

- **Food composition:** Choosing raw, organic (when possible), and whole foods over processed foods and sugar drinks.

- **Supplements:** Choosing a supplement only after researching its effects, chemical makeup and provider.

TOP 10 GUIDELINES FOR SPORTS NUTRITION

1. **Eat every 2–4 hours.** You do not need a full meal every three hours, but eating more often will help you meet your daily calorie demands, stabilize your blood sugar, ensure adequate recovery, and help you maintain a better body composition.

2. **Include complete, lean protein each time you eat.** Protein is muscle food, and muscle does not build itself. You must feed your muscles multiple times each day. It's not necessarily easy to get enough protein, but it's manageable if you have some with each meal.

3. **Eat vegetables every time you eat.** Vegetables provide the vitamins and minerals responsible for your body's high performance and recovery. The easiest way to do this is to have some veggies every time you eat.

4. **Focus on carbohydrate timing.** Simple carbs post-workout and complex carbs pre-workout and in your remaining meals. See the Glycemic Index on page 48.

5. **Do not be afraid of healthy fats.** There are three types of fat: saturated, mono-unsaturated and polyunsaturated. Eating all three kinds in a healthy balance can dramatically improve your health and even help you lose body fat.

6. **Drink mostly zero calorie drinks.** The best choices are water and green tea. Obviously, this rule can be broken in moderation, but the more high calorie beverages you consume, the harder it is going to be to become leaner. A leaner athlete is a faster athlete.

7. **Focus on whole foods.** Eating whole foods is always better than taking supplement powders or pills. Try to eat as much whole food protein, vegetables and fats as you can. If you need a little extra to get you where you need to be, then supplement with protein powders, fiber and fish oil.

8. **Develop food preparation strategies.** The hardest part about eating well is making sure you can follow the previous seven guidelines consistently. And this is where preparation comes in: you might know what to eat, but if isn't available, you'll blow it when it's time for a meal. Recall our discussion of PREPARE from Mental Toughness on page 10.

9. **Introduce a healthy variety only after you have developed a routine.** Healthy eating doesn't have to be boring or bland, but kids your age need to develop a consistent routine before introducing variety. Master the basics first.

10. **Be a high school kid once in a while!** The above guidelines may seem like they will be impossible to follow all the time, and that's honestly true. Are you never going to have pizza, soda, or your favorite treats ever again? Of course not! However, at this age, the development of healthy habits is a life skill that will pay dividends far beyond baseball. So plan on breaking the rules…but only about 10 percent of the time.

HEALTH AND PERFORMANCE CHECKLIST

Before you read on, test yourself to see where you are with your nutrition. Remember to answer honestly; honest efforts yield honest results.

Give yourself 1 point for each question you answer YES to:

☐ Do you eat breakfast seven days a week?

☐ Do you eat foods from at least three different food groups at breakfast?

☐ Do you eat three balanced meals at approximately the same time each day?

☐ Do you eat a nutritious mid-morning and mid-afternoon snack?

☐ Do you eat at least three pieces of fresh fruit each day?

☐ Do you eat at least five servings of fresh vegetables each day?

☐ Do you choose primarily high fiber breads and cereals?

☐ Do you eat lean and/or low-fat protein at each meal?

☐ Do you limit your intake of saturated fat (found in meats, cheeses, dairy products, butter)?

☐ Do you eat at least two servings of "good fat" each day (found in nuts, seeds, extra virgin olive oil, olives, avocados, fish, and/or eggs)?

☐ Do you limit your intake of processed and refined foods (foods made from white flour, foods high in sugar and sodium, packaged foods)?

☐ Do you eat and drink adequately to maintain your body weight?

☐ Do you eat a post-workout or post-practice snack within 30 minutes of completion?

☐ Do you eat a healthy post-workout or post-practice meal within two hours?

☐ Do you sleep at least 7–8 hours each night?

☐ Do you go to bed at approximately the same time each night and get up at approximately the same time each morning?

☐ Do you research and choose supplements based on third party organizations that test dietary supplements for safety?

SCORE: _____

> **14–17:** Performing like a champ!
> **9–13:** Losing an edge!
> **< 9:** Missing out big time!

EATING ACCORDING TO YOUR BODY TYPE

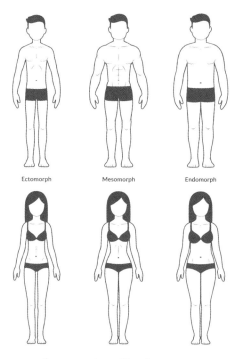

There are three general categories of body types: **ectomorph**, **mesomorph** and **endomorph.**

Ectomorph

- Runner or endurance athlete build (think skinny high school baseball player)
- Can handle a higher carb diet
- Fast metabolism, or "hard gainer"
- Best diet strategy may be higher carb and lower fat

Mesomorph

- Football linebacker build or high level wrestler, 182/195 weight class, or Mike Trout
- Can handle a medium carb diet
- Builds muscle easier than most
- Best diet strategy may be a balance of carbs, lean protein, and healthy fat

Endomorph

- Larger build with excess body weight in the belly and hips (think of the catcher from "The Sandlot")
- Poor carbohydrate tolerance
- Slower metabolism and difficulty with weight loss
- Best diet strategy may be most carbs from fruits and vegetables, high protein and medium fat

High school bodies are often a combination of these characteristics because you are still physically maturing, but the vast majority of high school baseball players are looking to add weight and muscle. Allow your body to be your guide by experimenting with different nutritional approaches until you find what works best. Ultimately, honest efforts will yield honest results.

PRE- AND POST-EXERCISE NUTRITION

A thletes need to eat before any strenuous physical activity or competition—that much should be obvious. But what might be less obvious, particularly to younger athletes, is the need to refuel and rehydrate after exercise. Eating properly at each stage of physical activity and providing your body with the fuel it needs to succeed is a critical part of developing as an athlete and is one of the easiest ways to set yourself up for victory…or defeat.

PRE-EXERCISE NUTRITION

Making sure that athletes are properly fueled before any workout, practice, tournament or game is crucial to ensuring good performance and avoiding unnecessary injury or fatigue. Eating a meal high in carbohydrates raises blood glucose levels, which the muscles then make use of (rather than depleting their own glycogen stores for energy), which in turn saves that glycogen for exercise.

For this reason, it's important that you eat breakfast prior to exercise to replenish muscle and liver glycogen stores after the overnight fast. A large meal should be eaten **3–4 hours prior to any physical event.** This allows for maximum digestion, absorption, and metabolism of the nutrients while also ensuring that your stomach has emptied prior to the event.

Carbohydrates

Carbohydrates are an important source of fuel for the body. Carbs are digested and absorbed quickly by the muscles as glucose, sparing muscle glycogen for exercise. Carbohydrates are the primary source of energy for anaerobic and prolonged high intensity aerobic activity. It also costs the body less energy to digest carbohydrates than protein or fat, which saves energy for your sport.

Look for carbohydrates that are easy to digest and have a low to moderate fiber content. **Low glycemic index carbohydrates may be best** in order to avoid a spike in blood sugar and which can aid in fueling the body for prolonged exercise. Examples include spaghetti, wheat, rye or pumpernickel bread, banana, apple, pears, grapefruit, oranges, strawberries, carrots and peas.

Fluids

It is critical to hydrate and prevent dehydration from occurring too soon during exercise. To aid this, 17–20 ounces of hydrating fluids should be consumed 2–3 hours before a practice or competition, as well as 7–10 ounces after the warm-up, 10-15 minutes before practice/competition.

For more information on staying properly hydrated, see page 41.

Protein and Fat

Players should reduce their consumption of both fats and proteins prior to an event. Both of these digest slowly and require a higher metabolism for digestion and absorption. The additional metabolic heat generated by this process may also impair performance in hot weather. On top of that, having too much protein or fat in your digestive system can prevent carbohydrates from quick digestion and absorption to the muscles.

Instead, aim **to consume a small amount of lean protein in your pre-exercise meal.** This will provide a small amount of energy to muscle cells, decrease the breakdown of muscle protein, increase protein synthesis in muscle after the workout, and delay hunger prior to the exercise.

A good place to start is a fist-sized piece of chicken, turkey, egg whites, pork, or ham. Try to avoid nuts, seeds, high-fat cuts of meat, and full-fat dairy prior to a competition or workout.

Fiber

Having too much fiber in your pre-competition meal can lead to **gastric distress** during the competition/activity. Fiber also **decreases the**

absorption of glucose and delays gastric emptying. For this reason, players should avoid raw vegetables and high bran cereal, as well as high fructose-based drinks.

Sugar and Caffeine

It can be tempting to go for that sugary soda or caffeinated beverage before a big game to give a player an extra boost of energy. And while they can produce the desired effect, it's best to limit these to at least an hour before any exercise. High sugar content may cause gastric distress when not given proper time to be absorbed prior to a workout, and caffeine can cause gastro-intestinal distress. Finally, energy gained from pre-workout and caffeine drinks does not last. The last thing you want as a player is to "crash" in the fourth or fifth inning.

POST-EXERCISE NUTRITION

These are the "Three Rs" of post-exercise nutrition:

1. Refuel
2. Rehydrate
3. Repair

Refueling, **rehydrating**, and allowing your muscles time and material to **repair** themselves after every lift, practice or game ensures that the player is "triggering" the right adaptations for optimal recovery and physical improvement.

And this goes for everyone—athletes who engage in regular intense exercise, athletes who play in tournament competitions or multiple qualifying round sports, and especially those who are involved in competitive events/sports with only 1–2 days for recovery. Everyone's bodies need proper support after exercise to repair and replenish.

When should I eat?

The short answer is, **immediately!** However, the "window of opportunity" for optimal post-exercise nutrition is in the first two hours post-exercise, when the rate of carbohydrate storage in the muscles is at its peak. Eat small meals consisting mainly of carbs and some protein every 2-3 hours.

What should I eat?

First, carbohydrates. Replenishing your carb stores is vital to the recovery process and necessary for optimal energy levels during future workouts. Eat within the first 15 minutes of ending an exercise to initiate replenishment of carb stores (glycogen) within the muscles. You play an endurance based sport, sometimes playing multiple games in a day—continue to eat/drink 200-300 calories of carbs every 2 hours after exercise to give the body a steady stream of carbs, allowing for optimal replacement of used stores.

    Second, protein. "Feeding" your muscles with the necessary building materials helps stimulate muscle repair and growth, and aids in the replenishment of glycogen when paired with carbohydrates. Consume proteins within 1 hour of activity.

    Third, fluids. Drink, even if you are not thirsty. For every pound of sweat loss through activity, you should be drinking 16 ounces of water. Fluids with sodium, potassium, and magnesium content will help speed up rehydration. This goes double for my catchers out there, after catching a double header!

MUSCLE GAIN VS. BODY FAT LOSS FOODS

When it comes to gaining muscle while burning fat, remember that total calories dictates everything. Any food can be considered viable for a "muscle gain" or "body fat loss" plan, in the context of your total diet. If you are operating at a calorie deficit trying to lose body fat, then the food you eat is considered usable for body fat loss. If you are eating more calories trying to gain muscle, then the food you eat is good for "muscle gain."

    With that said, there are foods that lend themselves more easily to muscle gain and body fat loss, which are detailed in the next sections.

USING NUTRITION TO PREVENT MUSCLE CRAMPING

First, what is a muscle cramp? Any athlete is familiar with these; a muscle cramp is a painful, involuntary skeletal muscle contraction that will not relax. Athletes get muscle cramps for a number of reasons:

- Dehydration, as a large loss of water and electrolytes can lead to muscle cramps

- A lack of minerals in food or drinks

- Muscle fatigue due to inadequate training

While that last one, muscle fatigue from inadequate training, can only be corrected by revising one's training plan, there are a number of ways to avoid muscle cramps from other causes through proper nutrition:

- Sip plenty of fluids before, during, and after exercise. While exercising in the heat or for longer than 30 minutes, grab an electrolyte enhanced beverage, like a sports drink.

- Eat foods high in electrolytes and minerals. Minerals to target include calcium (through sources like spinach, kale, turnips, collard greens, and dairy products) and magnesium (through sources like nuts, green leafy vegetables, milk and meat).

- Stretch before exercise, and increase the intensity and duration of your exercise gradually, as your body allows for it.

- Salt your foods with sea salt to fulfill your body's sodium needs, as opposed to processed table salt.

FUELING YOUR BODY FOR ALL-DAY TOURNAMENTS

Today is the showcase tournament. Your travel team tournament. College coaches will be watching. You have multiple games in one day that could shape your baseball future.

For those involved in youth sports, every season usually includes at least multiple tournaments. After dedicating so much time and energy to practice, it's important not to burn out during these long weekends due to improper nutrition and relying on the awful options at the local snack stands. Having a pre-planned nutrition plan ensures that the energy to achieve peak performance is there when you need it.

Rather than spend money on unhealthy foods at the concession stand that could hinder performance, prepare a "tournament cooler" using these quick, easy-to-follow suggestions:

- **Keep it safe.** Do not introduce any new foods. Doing so may bring about intestinal distress.

- **Keep it simple.** Focus on easily digestible and appetizing foods in-between games, including low-fat granola bars, fresh fruit, low-fat yogurt, nut butter sandwiches, trail mix, string cheese and low-fat chocolate milk.

- **Keep hydrated.** Dehydration is the quickest way to derail your performance over the course of one day and multiple games. For every pound of weight lost, drink 22 ounces of a sports drink or water. You can even take a bathroom scale to the tournament to keep track of your body weight throughout the day.

GAINING MUSCLE

Strength can easily separate two players of similar skill levels. A skilled but weak hitter can make contact but only hit singles; a skilled and *strong* hitter can make contact and drive the ball into the gaps or over the fence. This strong and fast rule is the reason high school players are constantly striving for more strength and speed to give them an edge. The results speak for themselves: just look at the difference between a junior varsity (JV) and a varsity athlete's body playing the same position. Talent aside, the biggest difference between a varsity and a JV player is strength, power, and speed. Gaining muscle contributes to all three of these advantages.

MUSCLE GAIN STRATEGIES

Eat More

Increasing caloric consumption combined with an exercise program targeting specific muscle groups leads to an increase in muscle mass in those areas. You especially need to increase the number of calories you eat on heavy activity days. **If you want to increase lean muscle, the number of calories you eat must exceed the number of calories burned during exercise.** You must take in enough calories to meet the physical demands of your day-to-day activities. If not, the body is forced to sacrifice lean muscle tissue for energy.

But how much more should you be eating? As a general rule, look to eat 500–700 more calories than what you are currently eating. Of those 500–700 calories, **50 percent should be carbohydrates, and 50 percent should be from protein sources.**

Put even simpler: add another 1–2 portions of carbohydrate and protein each day. For example, a peanut butter and jelly sandwich and a glass of milk, or a turkey and cheese sandwich with a banana and chocolate milk, would work well to fulfill both requirements.

Follow a Nutrient-Dense Diet

Dairy products, vegetables, fruit, beans, meat, and grains all have their place in your diet. Eating from only a few of the available food groups doesn't provide your body with all the nutrients that you need to perform at maximum capacity.

Snack Strategically

To help hit all the target food groups, as well as help boost your total caloric intake, you should make a point of snacking throughout the day. Fruit, nuts, Greek yogurt, whey protein shakes, and nutrition bars are all great options to help support a muscle-building diet.

You should also eat a snack post-workout, and eat no more than 2 hours after exercise. This snack should be both carbohydrate- and protein-rich; the carbohydrates restore your used muscle energy stores while the protein stimulates muscle repair and growth.

Finally, eat snacks before bedtime! Eaten one hour before sleep, nutrient dense snacks like a sandwich with milk, protein bar, or leftovers from dinner will help ensure your body has everything it needs while it works on repairing your damaged muscle tissue overnight.

Below, you'll find a list of the food groups (and examples of each) that can best benefit muscle growth. However, none of these foods are a miracle overnight muscle maker. Muscle growth is a slow process—expect to see no more than a half-pound to a pound of muscle growth a week, when consuming extra calories (combined with weight training).

MUSCLE GAIN FOODS

Lean beef. On average, a three-ounce serving of lean beef is only 154 calories, yet it provides ten essential nutrients, including iron, zinc and B-vitamins. More importantly, it provides your body with high quality protein (remember, not all proteins are equal), and a high level of amino acid that works with insulin to promote muscle growth.

Milk. Milk is high in protein, carbohydrates, Vitamins D, A, and calcium, and is an easy way to take in the extra calories for muscle growth. Chocolate milk is highest in calories!

Oatmeal. Oatmeal is an ideal source of carbs due to both its low glycemic index (GI) value and the fact it is minimally processed.

Sandwiches. Peanut butter and honey sandwiches make for an excellent snack. Add an extra piece of cheese to your turkey or ham sandwich for an extra 115 calories. Make it a triple-decker sandwich with an extra slice of bread, and you've got a nutrient-dense meal.

Lean protein. Chicken, eggs, fish, pork, beans, and red meat are all great examples of lean protein.

Cottage cheese. Few people know this, but cottage cheese is constituted from relatively pure casein protein—a slow-digesting protein, which means it is perfect for muscle recovery.

Salad. Pile on the vegetables and protein choices like beans, eggs, ham, and cheese to ensure a proper calorie count.

Pasta. Pasta is very rich in energy, and when combined with meat sauce, a pasta meal contains ingredients from three food groups: meat, grain and vegetable.

Healthy fats. I know some shudder at the thought of consuming fats, but good fats are essential for muscle growth. In fact, they play an essential role in the production of hormones (testosterone and growth hormones in particular) that are responsible for muscle growth and strength gains. Add a tablespoon of **olive oil** to your pasta or salads for an extra 120 calories.

Eggs. Eggs contain high quality protein, nine essential amino acids, choline, the right kind of fat, and vitamin D. To put it simply, they are the best value for your money.

Peanut butter. Two tablespoons of peanut butter makes up a whopping 190 calories! Buy organic, if possible, and avoid brands that add lots of sugar.

BURNING BODY FAT

A leaner athlete is a faster athlete. Compare any two athletes with a similar squat strength. If one has a higher body fat content than the other, who is faster?

The answer is the athlete with the lower body fat, simply due to having less body weight to move around. Today's game of baseball calls for better athletes than it did 10 years ago. If two players are of similar talent and skill, who gets the scholarship offers? The athletic and fit player who can potentially play different positions and shows the discipline and motivation to grow their body? Or the player who carries some extra weight around?

The answer should be obvious.

BODY FAT LOSS STRATEGIES
Eat Less Junk

If your goal is to burn body fat, start by eating less of what you know is bad for you—sugary drinks, sugary cereals, and unhealthy snacks. First, it is very important to create baseline. Rather than trying to count calories, keep an honest food journal for one week. Get on the scale weekly and measure the circumference of your belly at the belly button biweekly. Adjust your food based on the previous week's results. In addition, never skip meals to try and decrease calories. When you skip a meal, you'll see lowered energy levels during exercise; any muscle you've built will be cannibalized by the body for energy; and you run the risk of overeating later, leading to an unhealthy calorie balance.

Eat Healthier

Cutting out the junk is only the first part. If the entirety of your calorie consumption comes from junk food and sugary beverages, it doesn't matter how much you work out—you won't get the body you're looking for.

When creating a healthier lifestyle, follow these guidelines:

Cut out unhealthy fats. Cut any full fat items from your diet and replace them with healthy food choices to ensure your body uses up its current fat stores.

Avoid processed foods and "snack foods" like chips or pretzels.

Do not fry foods in oil or fat. Instead, opt to bake, broil, sauté, or microwave foods.

Eat plenty of vegetables throughout the day.

Increase dietary fiber to help satisfy hunger. By choosing whole wheat breads, fruits, and vegetables, you'll feel fuller while eating less.

Increase your water intake. Increasing your water intake up to 1 ounce per half pound of body weight will decrease hunger and help flush out your system.

Eat high-quality proteins that are low in fat. Lean ground meat, chicken, turkey, pork, ham, Canadian bacon, fish, eggs, and skim milk are all great options for low-fat, high value protein.

Eat smaller food portions. By decreasing the amount you eat at meals by 25 percent, you will decrease the number of calories you eat by…25 percent!

Eat slowly. It takes time for your body to sense that it is full. Eat slower, to help prevent overeating.

On the next page, you'll find a list of foods that can help in a fat burning diet. Please remember, however, that losing weight is a slow process, one requiring a daily awareness of calorie intake and expenditure. It's just like balancing a budget. You should expect to see results on a weekly basis, but only in the 0.5–2-pound range for most players. Players who are 225–250 lbs. can afford to lose 2–4 pounds per week. This is the ideal balance to maximize fat loss and minimize muscle loss.

BODY FAT LOSS FOODS

Beverages. Prefer skim milk over whole or chocolate milk, and drink water rather than sports drinks or sugary juice at meals.

Grains. Eat plain whole-grain toast without jam or butter. Prefer whole grains, as their fiber content keeps you feeling fuller, longer.

Dressings. Stay away from full fat and high sugar salad dressings, using extra virgin olive oil with balsamic vinegar instead. A poor choice in dressings can quickly ruin a healthy salad.

Snacks. Fruits and vegetables make for excellent snacks. They are higher in fiber (which will help keep you full), low in fat and calories, and can be eaten fresh or frozen. Protein bars with minimal ingredients are also great choices. Reduce (or completely avoid) fried foods such as French fries or onion rings, and sweets like cakes, cookies and ice cream.

Low-fat meats. Choose low-fat meats like chicken or turkey instead of bacon, sausage, or pepperoni.

Soup. Prefer broth-based soup instead of creamy soups; soup in general is great because the high water content fills you up and keeps you hydrated.

THE GLYCEMIC INDEX

It is beyond the scope of this book to break down completely the glycemic index; thankfully, there are entire books dedicated to the subject. To briefly summarize, the glycemic index is a simple rating system that measures how quickly carbohydrates are broken down into glucose and enter the blood stream.

High Glycemic Index

These are foods that are quickly converted to energy, and just as quickly used up. These "simple carbs" make for a short-term energy source and are therefore perfect for post workout athletes as a way to accelerate recovery after a grueling workout.

Examples include white bread, high sugar cereals, and white rice.

Low Glycemic Index

These are foods that are slower to break down into energy, and make for a long-term fuel source. These "complex carbs" should make up the majority of an athlete's carbohydrate consumption, especially those who are trying to lose body fat in the off season.

Examples of complex carbs include brown rice, Ezekiel bread, steel cut oatmeal, and most vegetables.

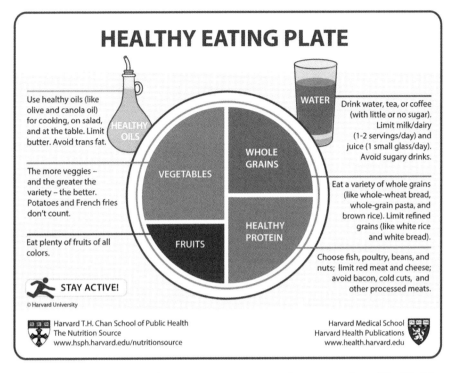

HEALTHY EATING PLATE

Use healthy oils (like olive and canola oil) for cooking, on salad, and at the table. Limit butter. Avoid trans fat.

WATER Drink water, tea, or coffee (with little or no sugar). Limit milk/dairy (1-2 servings/day) and juice (1 small glass/day). Avoid sugary drinks.

The more veggies – and the greater the variety – the better. Potatoes and French fries don't count.

Eat a variety of whole grains (like whole-wheat bread, whole-grain pasta, and brown rice). Limit refined grains (like white rice and white bread).

Eat plenty of fruits of all colors.

Choose fish, poultry, beans, and nuts; limit red meat and cheese; avoid bacon, cold cuts, and other processed meats.

STAY ACTIVE!

© Harvard University

Harvard T.H. Chan School of Public Health
The Nutrition Source
www.hsph.harvard.edu/nutritionsource

Harvard Medical School
Harvard Health Publications
www.health.harvard.edu

Copyright © 2011, Harvard University. For more information about The Healthy Eating Plate, please see The Nutrition Source, Department of Nutrition, Harvard School of Public Health, www.thenutritionsource.org, and Harvard Health Publications, www.health.harvard.edu.

HYDRATION

Staying hydrated helps you fight fatigue, keep your mental focus, support the body during twice-a-day practices, stave off cramps, and boost recovery. Dehydration can range from mild to severe, with symptoms including dizziness or a lightheaded feeling, nausea or vomiting, muscle cramps, dry mouth, and a lack of sweating.

Common symptoms of dehydration include:

- Thirst

- Flushed skin

- Dizziness or lightheadedness

- Mental confusion

- Nausea, diarrhea, vomiting

- Heat sensations or chills

- Weakness

- Loss of consciousness

- Headache

- Risk for heat illness

- Risk factor for sickle cell trait or disease

- Risk factor for rhabdomyolysis

Dehydration will also lead to negative effects on both your athletic and cognitive abilities, causing your performance to worsen as the degree of dehydration increases. In a state of mild to moderate dehydration, for example (2-5% body mass deficit), you'll experience a decreased sweat rate, decreased cardiovascular performance, and a decrease in anaerobic performance—meaning less strength and power. This is in addition to the hit you'll take to cognitive functions like task performance, reaction time, short term memory and mood.

Once dehydration becomes severe (crossing the line over a 5% body mass deficit), you'll start to be at risk of maintaining your body's normal thermoregulatory function. This means an increased risk of potentially life-threatening heat illnesses like heat stroke, which in turn means a threat to vital organ function and an increase in exhaustion and fatigue.

Bottom line? *Stay hydrated.* Staying hydrated is one of the easiest ways for an athlete to increase their performance, whereas becoming dehydrated is one of the quickest ways to tank performance. Remember that cool fluids pull double duty in your system by helping to cool you down, while also leaving the stomach faster, allowing for better hydration

WHEN SHOULD YOU HYDRATE?

The short answer is "**often.**" Two hours before any exercise, you should look to drink at least 2 cups / 16 ounces / 1 bottle of water. Five to fifteen minutes before a workout, drink a further 1 cup (8 ounces) water. Every 10–15 minutes during a workout is another ½–1 cup of water, and each of these numbers only increases in hot weather—when exercising in a hot environment (such as a hot gym in the summertime), drink as often as possible to minimize fluid loss from sweating.

> **Attention to all coaches and players:** Athletic trainers or others supervising athletes should be aware of all signs/symptoms of dehydration: thirst, headache, dizziness, cramps, vomiting, nausea, weakness, etc.

Here are some tried-and-true rehydration strategies during athletic activity:

- **Carrying around a bottle of water** during the day makes it easier to stay hydrated.

- **Drink even if you are not thirsty.** Thirst is our body's way of saying that we are already dehydrated; do not rely on it as an indicator.

- **Sports drinks are great for long activities and during hot weather.** The carbs keep you energized while the fluids and electrolytes keep you hydrated. (Beverages should have sufficient sodium content.) Liquid I.V., BioSteel, and Pedalyte are my favorites.

- **Within 4 hours post-exercise,** replace about 150% of fluid loss, electrolytes, carbohydrates, and protein.

STAYING SAFE IN HOT TEMPERATURES

If you're going to be playing or practicing outside during the sweltering summer heat, or any other time when you're at increased risk of dehydration, it's important to take steps to ensure you're not burning yourself out. Completing a heat acclimatization period—gradually increasing your time in the heat—can be key to assisting your body in adjusting to the higher cooling demands of hotter temperatures. Be sure to maintain a proper water supply at all venues during practice/games.

And if you can, make use of a Wet Blub Globe Temperature (WBGT). These devices actually measure the heat stress in direct sunlight, which takes into account temperature, humidity, wind speed, sun angle and cloud cover (solar radiation). (This differs from the heat index, which takes into consideration temperature and humidity and is calculated for shady areas.) Having more information about just how punishing your practice or game space is going to be will help you better prepare to stay cool and hydrated.

Here's a fun fact: Caffeine does not compromise rehydration or increase urine output when consumed in small quantities.

And here's a not-so-fun fact: You can actually OVER hydrate. Too much water can lead to Exercise-Associated Hyponatremia (EAH), a potentially fatal condition caused by low sodium (salt) concentration in body water. EAH typically results from ingesting water beyond the level needed to replenish sweat loss.

DIETARY SUPPLEMENTS

Since dietary supplements are not regulated by the Food and Drug Administration (FDA), the safety of these supplements can always be compromised. As a result, third party organizations (Informed Choice, NSF Certified for Sport, the Banned Substance Control Group, and the Resource Exchange Center) test dietary supplements for safety.

However, these third-party organizations are checking primarily to make sure that what is listed on the label is actually in the bottle. For example, Red Bull has been tested as "safe," but that does not mean it is a good or safe choice for you to *drink*. It just means you are "safe" in that you can know what is inside the bottle or can.

For athletes who are interested in supplements, we recommend they start with the results of their Health and Performance Checklist (page 24). This assessment provides 17 healthy opportunities for an athlete to improve on their personal sports nutrition before turning to dietary supplements. This places the emphasis on developing healthy habits rather than taking shortcuts—a valuable life skill for younger, impressionable high school players.

For players (and parents of players) who insist on specific suggestions, the best option is to provide supplements from a third-party organization with rock solid research from research-based, peer-reviewed journals toward their safety and efficacy.

Working from that criterion, here are the "Top 4" that we recommend:

The Top 4

1. **Protein.** Either whey or casein, or a combination of both, to increase your daily protein intake and help muscle recovery.

2. **Fish oil.** To help heart health and muscles recovery.

3. **Creatine.** To add a few reps in the weight room and build strength.

4. **Fiber.** To help digestion and make a thicker smoothie.

As a bonus, **supplement Vitamin D3.** During the winter months (your very important off-season), you get less sunlight—your major source of Vitamin D3. Vitamin D3 can help fight off the hazards of cold and flu season, reduce muscle inflammation, stress, and general aches and pains.

PROTEIN

Why supplement with protein? Because sometimes it is simpler to drink a protein shake after a tough workout, rather than sitting down for a full meal. Diets higher in protein can help an athlete lose body fat if their total calories are in check.

There are two general classifications of protein supplements:

Concentrate. This is protein that is derived from various food sources and is "concentrated" by removing the non-protein parts, resulting in a protein that is 70–85 percent pure and a bit cheaper by cost.

Isolate. Taking the concentration process to the next step, "isolation" removes a much higher percentage of non-protein content. This process yields a protein that is up to 95% pure and is more expensive.

Different Types of Protein

Whey protein. Easily the most popular, whey protein is essentially the by-product of turning milk into cheese. Whey protein is the perfect post workout protein because it immediately breaks down after exercise due to its quick absorption rate.

Casein protein. The primary difference between casein and whey is that casein digests over a longer period of time. To get the best of both worlds, find a protein powder that mixes whey and casein for a day meal-replace-ment-type shake that keeps you fuller for longer.

Egg protein. Egg protein is a complete protein made by separating egg yolks and dehydrating the egg whites. Egg proteins are rich in vitamins and minerals. This is the most bioavailable form of protein powder, meaning you will digest nearly 100 percent of the egg protein powder you consume.

Plant-based. Plant-based is most often made from yellow split peas and is a popular protein source for vegetarians and vegans. As with most plant-based proteins, pea protein is hypoallergenic. Pea proteins have very few additives or artificial ingredients, making it the most similar to a whole-food source.

FISH OIL

Why supplement with fish oil? Simply put, because the standard American diet does not include eating wild caught fish 2–3 times per week. Fish oil can help reduce inflammation, and athletes who have lower levels of inflammation recover faster.

Different Types of Fish Oil

While there are a number of different varieties of fish oil available, the important thing is to find one that is suitably rich in two specific groups of omega-3 fatty acids known as docosahexaenoic acid (DHA) and eicosapentaenoic acid (EPA).

Look for supplements containing at least 1000mg of combined EPA and DHA per serving, coming from at least 50 percent of the total amount of fish oil per serving. You want to aim for a ratio of 3:2 of EPA to DHA.

Note: Current research shows no issue with taking fish oil supplements, except for those on blood thinning medications. Please consult your physician before introducing any new supplements into your diet.

CREATINE

Why supplement with creatine? Answer: because you cannot realistically eat 2–3 pounds of red meat every day. This costs you potential benefits, which you can avoid (while still eating healthfully) by incorporating creatine supplements.

Creatine is perhaps the most researched supplement on the market, yet is still often misunderstood. In fact, recent research shows creatine to be safe for men, women and children alike.

Here's how it works: supplementation can increase the body's phosphocreatine and creatine stores. More creatine means more potential ATP (adenosine triphosphate), which is what the body uses as an energy source for rapid and powerful movements lasting fewer than 10 seconds, such as short sprints or a heavy set of squats.

Creatine can enhance muscle recovery, enhance your tolerance for exercise in hot weather (due to improved water retention) and can boost recovery rates from injury by way of increased strength and muscle gains.

Different Types of Creatine

While there are a multitude of creatine supplements competing for your attention and business, creatine monohydrate is the only form you should be looking at. **Creatine monohydrate** has the benefit of being the most extensively studied and clinically effective form of creatine, according to the International Society of Sports Nutrition (ISSN). Look for a label that lists creatine monohydrate as its only ingredient.

FIBER

Why supplement with fiber? Because you probably don't eat enough vegetables, fruits, legumes, whole grains, nuts and seeds. Realistically, not many young athletes do.

Fiber is a non-digestible dietary material (think "roughage"). Diets higher in fiber tend to lead to leaner, more muscular athletes. When looking to add fiber to your diet, look for a label that lists "psyllium husk powder" as its only ingredient.

Different Types of Fiber

Soluble fibers. Viscous and fermentable, soluble fibers can lower blood cholesterol levels.

Insoluble fibers. These bulk up stool volume and help improve motility.

THE FINAL WORD ON DIETARY SUPPLEMENTS

Supplements can certainly help, but they are not magic. Focus on consistent healthy eating rather than any specific diet plan or supplement, and review the diagram on page 22 comparing magnitudes (calories in versus calories out, macronutrients, nutrient timing, food composition, and supplements. Supplements are a very small, albeit valuable piece of an athlete's sports nutrition puzzle. After all, they are called supplements for a reason: they're meant to *supplement* a well-rounded diet, not replace it.

COACHING PLAYERS AND SUPPLEMENTS

A coach's policy must always be to educate players on the use of dietary supplements, not to endorse any specific usage. Players will always ask questions like, "What should I take?" or "Coach, what do *you* take?" Do not underestimate the influence you have on your player's lives. If they see what is in your training bag, or you tell them what you are taking, they will immediately head off to pick it up for themselves.

That said, you *should* provide your players and their parents with the resources to make safe, sound decisions. As soon as my players tell me they want to look into taking supplements, as well as why they want to, I bring the parents in (so we can all be on the same page). I give the parents some easy-to-read research, answer follow-up questions, and provide them with everything they need—while allowing them to make their own decisions.

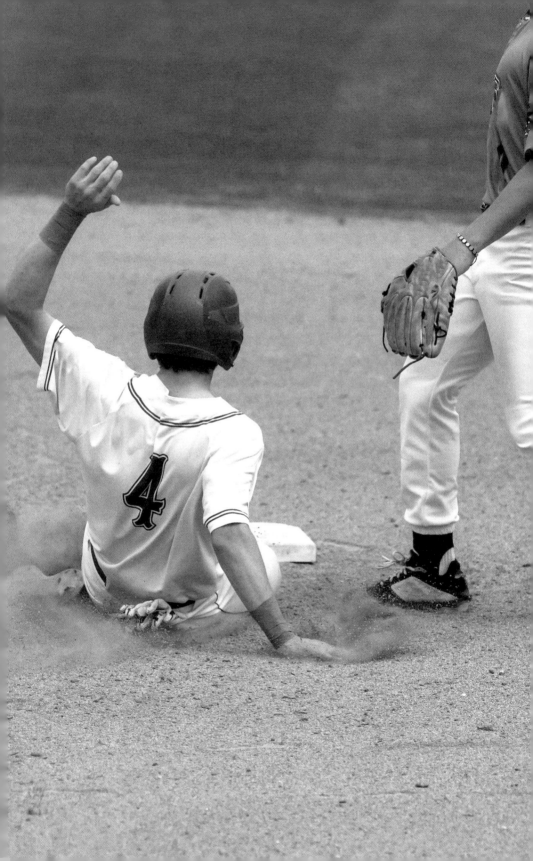

PART III: TRAINING

The best training programs follow principles. Just as in life, you must stay focused to be successful.

The following principles are found in the most successful training programs, and should serve as the foundation for any training regimen you institute.

Planned Performance Training. We use alternating periods of progressive overload and muscle regeneration as a way to maximize performance. Progressive overload refers to the gradual increasing of volume (reps × sets) and intensity (percentage of max) from workout to workout, or week to week. Muscle regeneration means allowing the body to recover from exercise. Things like recovery weeks (weeks of low volume, low intensity weight training), post-workout and post-game meals (composed of high carbohydrate/moderate protein content), foam rolling, pool mobility workouts, and many more, allow for proper recovery in between strenuous workouts.

Technique and Assessment. Teaching proper technique and assessing for competence are at the core of a coach's job. Through the course of teaching proper technique, we test for muscle imbalances and add corrective exercises to personalize workouts as needed.

Specificity. Workouts must be specific to an athlete's abilities, needs, goals, position, injury history, and training history.

Training Variety. A good training program incorporates a variety of different techniques to change up the routine and prevent athletes from losing motivation or plateauing. These include different methodologies like super sets and circuit training, as well as different equipment, like barbells, dumbbells, kettlebells, sandbags, and the slideboard.

Competition. To increase the energy of each student athlete, a balanced training program employs competition through various workout challenges. This keeps each athlete striving to improve, and provides them with the opportunity to take pride in their accomplishments.

Balanced Programming. A good program is one which incorporates all the basic movements found both on the field and in life into every workout. These include Upper Body Pull (horizontal and vertical), Upper Body Push (horizontal and vertical), Lower Body Pull, Lower Body Push, Lunge (Single Leg Strength), and Core Rotation and Stabilization.

Discipline and Motivation. This is something I picked up from 5/3/1 creator, Jim Wendler—understanding the difference between discipline and motivation. Discipline is internal: it's all about positive action, effort, habits, creating consistency, and getting your work done no matter what; it's about giving your best effort when nobody is looking. Motivation, on the other hand, is external. It's driven by emotions, which have ups and downs and lack consistency. Motivation means giving your best effort only after a coach or teammate tells you to. Making full use of them both—and understanding the limitations of each—are essential for any training plan to survive first contact with a living, breathing human athlete.

Remember: consistent hard work beats any workout program done inconsistently. The dirty secret to training high school athletes is that any program will work if done consistently. There's no need to scour YouTube for cutting edge programs or mimic what your favorite MLB players are doing. Stay true to the workouts laid out in this book and reach your truest potential!

Working from these training principles, we see the best training programs and workouts created. In the following section, we'll look at how best to incorporate these principles into both your program structure and the instruction and guidance you offer your athletes.

BASEBALL TRAINING

The game of baseball is primarily comprised of repeated, short, maximum-intensity bouts of sprints in the outfield, first steps for base stealers and infielders, powerful rotations for the hitter, and throws for the pitcher. Think about it: how many close plays do you see per game on first base decided by inches? For this reason, the ability to generate force, change direction, and rapidly decelerate tends to be the determining factor between victory and defeat in baseball. The diagram below does a great job showing multiple athletic movements in most sports.

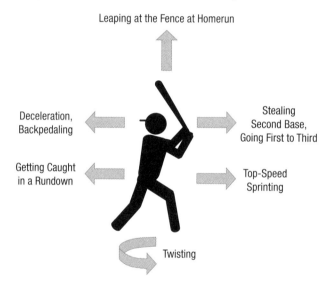

The 6 Load Vectors in Sports

The game of baseball includes the following movements:

- Vertical and horizontal jumps

- Lateral movement

- Change of direction (cutting)

- Acceleration and top-speed sprint

- Twisting and rotation

Therefore, the focus of any baseball training program, bearing in mind the physical demands and primary movements of baseball, should be on:

1. Stabilization and deceleration training to improve your ability to change directions and prevent ACL tears

2. Muscular strength and power with a focus on lateral glute strength, groin strength, and single leg training

3. Aerobic/anaerobic capacity and power for better conditioning

4. Acceleration development for a faster first step

5. Change of direction development

6. Reactive agility training (change of pace movements, responding to audio/visual cues)

7. Multi-movement agility combinations

8. Mobility to help prevent injury and to improve exercise technique

9. Sports nutrition to help daily recovery and build muscle

10. Rest and recovery to allow for healthy growth from strenuous workouts

ADDITIONAL FACTORS TO CONSIDER WHEN CREATING A PROGRAM

The workouts in this book are presented as "best case scenario" workouts, to be performed under ideal conditions. But there are many factors that can affect how you program:

- Do you have enough racks to allow your entire team to train at once?

- Do you have the staff/coaching to ensure proper technique during high skill exercises?

- Does your facility only have support stations, due to limited space and equipment?

- Do you have access to a field? To a track?

Every coach's facility is different, which is another reason why any "one-size-fits-all" college strength and conditioning program probably isn't going to work best in *your* facility.

THE IMPORTANCE OF SINGLE LEG TRAINING

The importance of single leg training with regards to your body's ability to jump, run, change directions, transition power, and prevent ACL tears cannot be overstated. When only one foot is in contact with the ground, your ankle is working overtime. To a lesser degree, the ankle also works to stabilize the rest of the body when in a staggered stance (like lunges or Bulgarian squats).

Learning to stabilize the ankle, knees, hips, and core all directly relate to improved athleticism. Add to that any change of direction and jumping off a single leg, and you'll find that building equal strength in each leg is essential to your development as a player.

Baseball is essentially a single leg power sport. Think about it—every player starts on two feet and transitions to one foot during every play:

- A third basemen starts in a ground ball position but has to dive to his left by pushing off his right foot.
- A pitcher goes into his wind-up or from the stretch and drives off his back leg, violently transitioning all his weight onto his front leg.
- Every hitter has some sort of leg kick, and in today's game, the leg kick is only getting bigger, further showing the importance of transitioning power from the back leg to the front leg.

On top of this, the need for improved hip mobility has never been greater. As a high school student, you likely sit for most of the day. During this time, your hips get tight. Any time you split your feet in the weight room (lunges, split squats, Bulgarian squats), you are working on your hip mobility.

BOYS VS. GIRLS: BASEBALL VS. SOFTBALL WORKOUT CONSIDERATIONS

There are a few crucial distinctions to consider when planning a training regimen for female athletes, as compared to male athletes. Programming around these differences will help ensure consistent progress in your players and prevent unnecessary frustration or injury.

1. Strength training is just as important for girls as for boys.

The first step I take in alleviating any fears my female players have about weight training is to teach them the reasons why heavy weights will not, cannot not, and do not "bulk them up." This is simply because women do not have nearly as much testosterone as men. Testosterone and muscle building potential are tightly linked, and because men have so much more testosterone (about 20 times more), they are better equipped to gain muscle. For this exact reason, women cannot get as big as men, no matter how much they lift, which is why I coach my girls to work harder (lift more weights) to build muscle.

You won't become "big" or "bulky" unless you're doing something illegal. Being big or bulky is a result of having bigger muscles with the same or worse body fat percentage. Most girls do not want that—they want toned, lean and athletic bodies.

A typical conversation might go like this:

> **Athlete:** "Coach Mike, lifting weight is for the boys. I only want to tone up my muscles so I'm going to stick to cardio."
> **Coach Mike:** "That's cool, but what does it mean to be 'toned'?"
> **Athlete:** "Leaner, less body fat…you know, more muscle definition."
> **Coach Mike:** "Great. Would you be more 'toned' with more or less muscle?"
> **Athlete:** "More."
> **Coach Mike:** "Which builds muscle, lifting weights or cardio?"
> **Athlete:** "…Weights, I guess."

2. Muscle size is a result of three factors, not a 15 lbs. dumbbell.

Increased muscle size results from the combination of three specific factors: a high volume of work, years of consistent training, and a surplus of calories.

It's important to understand that building muscle is not an overnight process. Many women think that if they start lifting weights, they'll wake up one morning and discover they're suddenly huge. This does not happen.

Muscles grow in proportion to the stimulus given. Lots of volume (4–6 sets for 3–4 exercises per muscle group), which is a traditional bodybuilding program, is designed to increase muscle size. Athlete programming designed for strength, power, and speed, as seen in this book, uses a lower volume with moderate to heavy weights to produce the desired effect.

Truly heavy weights (over 85% of your max) builds strength, not size. Remember, size is built with training volume (reps and sets). Working at over 85%, you simply cannot perform the number of sets and reps needed to build muscle size due to the stress it places on the body. On the flip side, the women you see (and whom young female athletes may admire) in magazines or on social media, doing sets of 10 with a weight they could easily lift 20 or 30 times without effort, are just wasting their time doing an exercise with a weight that makes no contribution to their fitness level or the development of muscle.

3. Most girls have little to no experience with lifting weights, especially the barbell.

Pay attention to and make use of the exercise progressions detailed in this book's program to allow girls time and space to learn the movements and build confidence. Girls leave their egos in the lockers, unlike boys; they are not looking for a 3-plate squat on the first day of workouts. Start them with body weight exercises, then build on top of those body weight exercises with dumbbells. Introduce the barbell only after the girls have started building some confidence in the weight room. (There are also some barbells designed specifically for female athletes, using specific grip patterns and bar widths, though these may not be available at all high school facilities.)

4. Female athletes are more prone to tearing their ACL.

The *Journal of Athletic Training* has published several research studies that show, when comparing sports that are played by both boys and girls, **girls are eight times more likely to suffer an ACL injury.**

The vast majority of ACL tears are non-contact, meaning they occur during planting and cutting movements with the knee collapsing inwards (valgus) and the leg at near full extension. Further, sudden or unexpected deceleration and changes of direction (think run downs), especially leaping in any direction outside their base of support (reaching for first base trying to beat out an infield single), creates a negative environment for the knee.

Additionally, as reported by the *American Journal of Sports Medicine*, girls have an approximately 1.6 times higher rate of injury per exposure than that of males in sex-comparable sports.

Instead of getting stuck on the numbers, let us focus on the whys of this trend, what we can do to mitigate risks, and what we can and cannot control.

First, why are girls more susceptible to the ACL tear? It's no secret that boys and girls are built differently, but the reasons for why the rate of ACL injuries are higher in girls is multifactored:

Hormones. Researchers have proposed that estrogen makes girls more vulnerable to ACL injury by weakening this ligament. It is possible that more ACL injuries in girls occur during the menstrual cycle when estrogen levels are high. During puberty, there is a sharp rise in estrogen levels, as well as growth spurts in the legs. Following one of these growth spurts, it takes time for the adolescent to develop good coordination with their newly elongated limbs. During these times of poor coordination, girls can be in poor landing, cut positions, which may potentially lead to more ACL tears.

Slower reflex times. The muscles stabilizing the knee may take a millisecond longer to respond in women than in men. Scientists suspect that this small difference in contraction time also leads to a higher rate of injury.

The intercondylar notch. This is the groove/tunnel in the femur through which the ACL passes, which is naturally smaller in women than in men. In addition, the ACL itself is smaller in women, which makes it more prone to injury.

Wider pelvis. Women typically have a wider pelvis as compared to the length of their legs, which makes the thigh bones angle downward more sharply than in men (this is called the Q angle). Therefore, more pressure is applied to the inside of the knee, creating a greater chance of valgus (knee collapsing in), which, in turn, can cause the ACL to tear. This is only amplified during landings and changes of direction.

More lax ligaments. Women's ligaments tend to have more "give" (laxity) than men. Excessive joint motion combined with increased flexibility may be a significant contributing factor.

The above are all constants—unchangeable factors related to being a female athlete. Thankfully, there are a number of things you can control to help reduce your chances of an ACL tear. These can be broken down into two categories, training based and non-training based. Here, we'll focus on the training based variables athletes, coaches, and parents can control.

Performing proper active warm-ups. While the days of static stretching are hopefully long behind us, I still have to remind varsity level sport coaches that their athletes must move and dynamically activate their muscles before they static stretch (if at all). See my Appendix A: Speed Development Playbook on GetFitNow.com for a full dynamic warm-up.

Learn to land properly. Girls often land flat-footed instead of on the balls of their feet after a jump. This improper landing puts pressure on the knee when the calf muscles should be absorbing the force. Training your body for proper landing is certainly something to work on as you better yourself athletically. I ask athletes to land like a cat – quietly and softly. I also tell them "I only want to see you land, I do not want to hear you land."

Core stability. Efficient core stability provides your legs with the ability to dynamically stabilize against abnormal forces (unpredicted deceleration, cuts, and landings). A "core" that activates properly allows the surrounding muscles to do their job by allowing a transfer of force. Poor core stability can indirectly set the stage for injury.

Develop improved hamstring strength. Girls typically have poor hamstring strength, which is considered one possible risk factor for ACL tears. If the hamstring cannot balance the power of the quadriceps (front thigh muscle), the imbalance can cause significant stress to the ACL, leading to injury. Therefore, you must strengthen the hamstring at the knee (leg curl variations) and at the hip (deadlift variations). These are both foundational exercises in this book's program.

Practice proper running posture. Women tend to run in a more upright position than men, adding stress to the ACL and resulting in less control over rotation of the knee joint when decelerating and changing directions. See my section on Jump Progression on page 86 for a full checklist on proper landings.

Develop each leg through single leg training. When a girl tears her ACL, the majority of her weight is on a single leg. While most athletes have a stronger leg, making them "right footed" or "left footed," girls tend to have a greater difference between legs in terms of muscle strength when compared to boys. Single leg strength is a foundational exercise in my program.

Develop improved quads strength. Studies have also shown that when girls hit puberty, they do not gain significant muscle mass in the quadriceps, whereas boys at the same stage do gain significant muscle mass. Therefore, girls have bigger, more mature bodies with less strength, putting them at an increased risk of ACL injury. That means girls must focus on increasing squat, deadlift, and lunge strength, all of which are foundational exercises in my program.

Observing proper rest, recovery, and downtime. An athlete's body can only get stronger and faster if given time to recover from the strenuous training and practice sessions. If you continue to work without proper recovery, you are setting your body up for potential injury.

NON-TRAINING BASED FACTORS

Entire books have been written on the non-training based factors that can potentially increase an athlete's chances of tearing an ACL. Suffice it say, I see four major factors that affect an athlete's physical development outside the weight room.

- **Increased AAU/travel games and practice.** Playing the same sport year round creates the potential for overuse.
- **Earlier specialization.** Not playing other sports at a younger age inhibits an athlete from developing foundational movement patterns in different directions.
- **Lack of free play.** Without free play, kids never develop the natural instincts, balance, and athleticism you see in other kids who were allowed to "play."
- **Unsupervised weight room workouts.** This could also be thought of as unqualified "strength" coaches teaching youth athletes; teaching young athletes improper technique, or advancing kids too quickly into high intensity/high volume plyometrics, increases their risk of injury and is criminal besides.

After reading that exhaustive list, here are the things you can focus on in the weight room to decrease your chances of an ACL tear:

- Improve ankle and hip mobility to get low ("Athletic or Ground Ball position") while changing directions
- Practice proper landing technique (double and single leg) to reduce force on the knee
- Build core stability to allow the body to function optimally
- Strengthen the lower body with a focus on single leg training and the posterior chain (glute and hamstrings) to develop deceleration strength

TIER 1 CORE LIFTS: MY "BIG 5"

A ny long-term program for the high school baseball athlete should be based on an exercise progression blueprint—one designed from the ground up to produce proficient movement and high strength levels in the core/foundation movements.

In this section, we will break down the basics of exercise progression and their rationale, using the Tier 1 or "Big 5" core lifts as examples. (The Workouts section of this book also includes programming for all of these exercises.)

My "Big 5"

1. Trap Bar Deadlift
2. Barbell Front Squat
3. Dumbbell Bench Press
4. Pull-Up/Chin-Up
5. Lunge

Strength training in baseball has evolved in the past 20 years. If you are a coach in your 40s and played baseball at any level (high school, college, or professional), you've probably heard that the bench press is bad for your shoulder, or that you should "never lift overhead."

These myths are starting to fade away as more research comes out, and young, progressive strength coaches are educating the next generation of players to take full advantage of the weight room.

This evolution in physicality is reflected in my "Big 5," which identifies the specific core lifts that best fit the typical athlete's physical needs at the high school level, their head coach's expectations, and the expectations placed on incoming college freshman.

Every exercise—every workout we do—is designed to help improve technical proficiency and the strength level of these "Big 5" foundational movements. Once mastered, my "Big 5" can lead any athlete into a truly advanced power program (dropping bombs), one which includes movements like the Olympic lifts (clean and snatch), back squat, and trap bar jump squat.

HOW TO USE THIS SECTION

In the following pages, we'll discuss in greater detail the "Big 5" movements. Because these exercises are so fundamental and foundational to the healthy development of movement and strength in high school athletes, each movement is explained with:

1. A step-by-step guide for athletes to help them build towards being able to successfully complete the target movement without difficulty.
2. A list of progression exercises for each movement. Think of these as "extra credit" exercises, ways to build from a well-established base and continue advancing the core movement.
3. Coaching points and helpful tips to allow athletes to feel confident as they master the basic movement and progress to its more difficult variations.

Tier 1 Core Lifts in the Workouts

These five exercises are the backbone and foundation of the varsity programs in this book, as well as the goal of the freshman and JV programs. At the varsity level, the Tier 1 core foundation movements are the focus during the in-season, off-season, and pre-season. Progression exercises #1, #2, and #3 (the exercises to the left of the Foundation Movements in the chart on pages 65–66 serve as the primary exercise for the varsity post-season program, to allow for active recovery in preparation for an intense off-season of training.

The exercises to the right of the foundation movements are progressions from the foundation movements—truly advanced exercises that focus on building strength and power. These are the impressive exercises you see professional and college players doing on social media. They are found primarily in the varsity post-season and pre-season programs.

PROGRESSION/ADVANCEMENT OF CORE LIFTS

Progression			Foundation Movements	Advancement		
#1	#2	#3		#1	#2	#3
Progression/Advancement of Tier 1 Core Lift						
Dumbbell or Kettlebell Goblet Squat	Kettlebell Sumo Deadlift	High Handle Trap Bar Deadlift	**Low Handle Trap Bar Deadlift**	Barbell RDL	Barbell Deadlift	Trap Bar Jump Squat
Body Weight Squat	Dumbbell or Kettlebell Goblet Squat	Barbell Front Box Squat	**Barbell Front Squat**	Barbell Front Pause Squat	Barbell Back Squat	Barbell Back Squat with Chains or Bands
Floor Push-Up series	Suspension Trainer Push-Up and/or Dips	Single Arm Dumbbell Bench Press	**Dumbbell Bench Press**	Swiss Barbell (Neutral Grip) Bench Press	Swiss Barbell (Neutral Grip) Close Grip Bench Press	Swiss Barbell (Neutral Grip) Close Grip Bench Press with Bands or Chains
Suspension Trainer Row	Pull-Up/ Chin-Up ISO Holds	Jumping Pull-Up/ Chin-Up with 3 ISO Hold	**Pull-Up/ Chin-Up**	Suspension Trainer Pull-Up	Weighted Pull-Up/ Chin-Up	Multi-grip Pull-Up/ Chin-Up Mechanical Drop Set
Body Weight Split Squat	Dumbbell Goblet Reverse Lunge	Single Leg Squat (standing on a bench or box)	**Lunge (Dumbbell Goblet Bulgarian Squat)**	Dumbbell Lateral Lunge	Dumbbell Skater Squat	Barbell Reverse or Walking Lunge
Progression/Advancement of the Tier 2 Core Lifts						
Drop Squat	Drop Split Squat	Depth Drop (off box)	**Jump (Squat Jump/Broad Jump)**	Weighted Squat Jump/ Broad Jump	Depth Drop Squat Jump	Continuous Hurdle Jumps
Single Arm Overhead Farmer Walk	Single Arm Front Rack Farmer Walk	Single Arm Farmer Walk	**Carry (Farmer Walk)**	Cross Body Farmer Carry	Heavy Trap Bar Farmer Walk	Heavy Trap Bar Single Arm Farmer Walk
Cable Lift	Cable Chop	Cable Pallof Press	**Rotate (Cable Rotation)**	Lunge Cable Lift/Chop/ Pallof Press	Medicine Ball Rotation Throw	Medicine Ball Lateral Hop Rotation Throw
Medicine Ball Scoop Throw	Medicine Ball Reverse Scoop Throw	Medicine Ball Acceleration Throw	**Throw (Medicine Ball Squat Press Throw)**	Medicine Ball Rapid Response Overhead Throw	Medicine Ball Rapid Response Linear Throw	Medicine Ball Rapid Response Lateral Throw

PROGRESSION/ADVANCEMENT OF CORE LIFTS

Wall drills and dynamic warm up for technique	Plyometric jumps for power and acceleration	Sled push for resisted speed and acceleration	Sprint	Change of direction/ speed	Reaction Agility Speed	Over Speed Training	
Core Stability PREP Program	Dead Bug Variations	Physioball Plank Circles	**Core Stability Suspension Trainer Plank Rollouts**	Ab Wheel Kneeling Rollouts	Single Arm Front Plank variations	Ab Wheel Pushup Rollouts	

Progression/Advancement of the Tier 3 Core Lifts

Glute Bridge	Single Leg Glute Bridge	Single Leg Hip Thrust	**Barbell Glute Bridge**	Barbell Hip Thrust	Kettlebell Single Leg Hip Thrust	3D Barbell Hip Thrust
Machine (Prone or Seated) Leg Curl	Physioball Leg Curl	Physioball Single Leg Curl	**Slider Leg Curl**	Slider Single Leg Curl	Glute Ham Raise	Nordic/ Russian Leg Curl
Banded Spanish Squat	Machine Leg Extension	Machine Single Leg Extension	**Backward Sled Pull**	Backward Sled Pull and Row	Lighter weights for Speed and Heavier Weights for Strength	Alternate Backward and Forward Sled Push
½ Kneeling Landmine or Dumbbell Press	Lunge Landmine or Dumbbell Press	Dumbbell Single Arm Shoulder Press	**Dumbbell Shoulder Press**	Barbell Z Press	Barbell Shoulder Press	Barbell Push Press
Suspension Trainer Row	Barbell Inverted Row	Dumbbell Supported Row	**Dumbbell One-Arm Row**	Dumbbell Row	Landmine Row	Barbell Row

The goal of this chart is to give athletes and coaches a clear and defined path to success. This is not a complete picture of all potential progressions and advancements available for these core movements; use this as a template to build from while preparing programs that are right for your athletes at their current level.

TRAINING BASEBALL PLAYERS: FOCUS POINTS

When training baseball players (pitchers included), we focus on the upper body, core, and throwing arm. But before we dive into the exercises that form the foundation of this program, a quick note on my upper body training philosophy as it relates to the baseball player. **Baseball players must be trained differently than other sports.** This isn't to say that you should treat them with kid gloves, mind you, but smarter training is needed for this specific sport. It is a highly skill-based sport, and throwing a baseball is a violent action that needs smart training to maintain injury-free throwing arms.

Baseball players can still be aggressive during their upper body training and ensure safe progress with a few simple adjustments. Start with the core stability section of the Progression/Advancement of Core Lifts table on page 65, as well as review the core stability section in the Tier 2 Core Lifts, found on page 66.

The following are some basic guidelines on where to focus training efforts for high school baseball players:

- Program more pulling exercises (row, chin-up, face pull) than pushing exercises (chest and shoulder press)

- Program more horizontal pull exercises (rows) than vertical pull exercises (chin-ups)

- Include neutral grip bench and shoulder press with dumbbells or Swiss bar/football bar

- Program multiple push-up variations for a healthy scapula

- Include a daily thoracic mobility routine (rotation and extension), one which features:
  - PVC Bench Thoracic Extension
  - Medicine Ball or Foam Roll Thoracic Extension
  - Kneeling Thoracic Rotations
  - Floor Medicine Ball Thoracic Rotations
  - Lunge Yoga Rotations

- Use a neutral or externally rotated grip (and avoid the pronated grip) whenever possible during as many upper body exercises as possible:
  - Band Pull-Aparts (with the palms up)
  - Dumbbell Shoulder Rear Delt Raise (with thumbs up)
  - Neutral Grip Pull-Ups
  - Rows (with a neutral grip)
  - Push-Ups (with neutral or slightly externally rotated hands on dumbbell handles)
  - If possible, use a safety bar for squats and the trap bar for deadlifts to reduce further stress on the shoulders
  - Use a neutral grip for *all* dumbbell pressing (bench and shoulder) exercises

- Practice daily band face pull variations before any pushing exercise.

- Place a greater emphasis on single arm and single leg training for greater core stability and balance.

TRAP BAR DEADLIFT

Requiring less lower back stress when compared to the traditional deadlift (due to a more vertical torso angle and the fact that your center of gravity stays inside the bar), the trap bar deadlift is a great way to quickly build confidence in younger athletes. The movement is easy to learn and allows the athlete to move some real weight; it also allows athletes who do not have the proper mobility for a traditional deadlift to deadlift safely.

Progression #1	Progression #2	Progression #3	Foundation Movements	Advancement #1	Advancement #2	Advancement #3
Dumbbell or Kettlebell Goblet Squat	Kettlebell Sumo Deadlift	High Handle Trap Bar Deadlift	**Low Handle Trap Bar Deadlift**	Barbell Deadlift	Barbell Deadlift and Sumo Deadlift	Trap Bar Jump Squat

COACHING POINT

The deadlift, which some call the hip hinge, is at once the most difficult and most important movement you can teach a young athlete. It is a challenging movement to coach and learn, but it can be picked up through patience, practice, and development of core stability strength. The deadlift/hinge movement directly relates to your athlete's speed development and power potential because it lays the proper foundation for the RDL and clean.

Building to the Trap Bar Deadlift

As I have become a more experienced coach, I have simplified the process I use to prepare athletes for the Trap Bar Deadlift. An athlete can be taught an acceptable High Handle Trap Bar Deadlift after only two exercises:

1. Dumbbell Goblet Squat
2. Kettlebell Sumo Deadlift

Both these exercises are low skill/high ROI. The Goblet Squat builds the requisite core and lower back strength needed in the deadlift, while the Kettlebell Sumo Deadlift allows an athlete to apply their new core strength to work on the hinge. No kettlebells available? Grab a dumbbell in a vertical grip as a substitute.

The key to all of this? **Strength standards.** Do you best to build your athletes up to 50 percent of their body weight in body exercises for 10–15 reps each. For example, your 145 lbs. sophomore short stop who is new to lifting should build up to a 70 or 75 lbs. Dumbbell Goblet Squat and Kettlebell Sumo Deadlift.

What If an athlete can Dumbbell Goblet Squat and Kettlebell Sumo Deadlift 50–60 percent of their body weight BUT still cannot properly hinge/deadlift? Wrap a strength band around their waist like a seatbelt and have it held behind with light tension to reinforce a "hips back" posture, which better loads the hamstrings.

But what about kettlebell swings? I hear you, I do, but I do **not** include the kettlebell swing in my progressions because I find too many coaches and players are doing it incorrectly: they are swinging the kettlebell but squatting up and down. A correct and effective kettlebell swing—one meant to learn and pattern the Hip Hinge (Deadlift), occurring at the hip with minimal knee bend (think RDL)—*is* a fantastic exercise. I certainly approve of Kettlebell Swings for athletes who are supervised by a certified strength and conditioning coach during their workouts.

Advancing from the Trap Bar Deadlift

1. Trap Bar RDL
2. Barbell Sumo Deadlift
3. Barbell Block Deadlift
4. Barbell RDL
5. Conventional Barbell Deadlift (from the floor)

TEACHING THE HANG CLEAN AND/OR POWER CLEAN

Once an athlete has reached a full bodyweight RDL and Front Squat, and a 1.5 times bodyweight high handle trap bar deadlift for 5 reps each, *and* has demonstrated proficiency in the catch positions (muscle clean and tall clean), only then do I advance them to the hang clean.

Whether your program is working towards the hang clean or power clean, the road to a successful clean focuses on two major areas: the Catch and the Pull.

I prefer a top-down approach when teaching the clean. I believe an athlete must be able to receive the bar before anything else. This teaches safe and proficient catches and emphasizes deceleration in younger athletes.

The Catch

Step 1: Muscle Clean
Goal: To practice receiving the barbell at the shoulders.
Execution: Pull the barbell from a mid-thigh position into a standing front squat rack position by aggressively shrugging your shoulders and punching your elbows up. Avoid jumping to better emphasize the front rack position.

Step 2: Tall Clean
Goal: To practice receiving the barbell at the shoulders while getting into the catch (front squat) position.
Execution: From a standing position and while on the balls of your feet, aggressively shrug your shoulders, punch your elbows forward, stomp your feet on the ground to pull yourself under the bar and into a proper catch position. You can practice catching in a quarter squat, half squat, or full squat position.

The Pull

Practice the following exercises to increase your athletes' speed with the barbell:
- Hang Clean Pull (Speed RDL)
- Hang Clean Jump Shrug
- Power Clean Pull (Speed Deadlift)
- Power Clean Jump Shrug
- Deadlift (with bands or chains)

Concurrently work in elements of the catch and the pull in order to build an athletic clean. Your athlete will present the ability to clean when they can properly execute a muscle clean (receiving the bar), front squat (catching the bar), and jump shrug (accelerating the bar).

Building Power and Vertical Jump with the Trap Bar Jump Squat

Some high school baseball players may never get to the level of hang clean, for a number of reasons. They may have preexisting wrist, elbow, or shoulder injuries, or they may lack the training time necessary to learn the requisite movements.

Enter the trap bar jump squat! This exercise checks all the boxes for power development, improved vertical jump, decreased pain at the elbow, wrist, and shoulder joints, and is an exercise most athletes can learn in minutes. Where hang cleans and power cleans are highly technical, requiring a significant investment of time to develop decent technique and can be tough on the wrists, elbows and shoulders, the trap bar jump squat allows for noticeable results even in less technically proficient student athletes.

BARBELL FRONT SQUAT

As a movement, the barbell front squat allows for more core activation and less lower back stress than the back squat. It's also great for younger, more inexperienced, and/or taller athletes, as less mobility at the ankle and hip is required to reach desired depths during the squat. It also promotes better posture and thoracic extension for the average student-athlete who sits for 6–8 hours a day, all while teaching the catch position of the clean.

Progres-sion #1	Progres-sion #2	Progres-sion #3	Foundation Movements	Advance-ment #1	Advance-ment #2	Advance-ment #3
Body Weight Squat	Dumbbell or Kettlebell Goblet Squat	Barbell Front Box Squat	**Barbell Front Squat**	Barbell Front Pause Squat	Barbell Back Squat	Barbell Back Squat with Chains or Bands

Building to the Barbell Front Squat

Use the following exercises as steppingstones to reach the ultimate goal of the perfectly executed barbell front squat.

1. Body Weight Box Squat
2. Body Weight Squat
3. Body Weight ISO Squat (work up to 20 second holds)
4. Dumbbell/Kettlebell Box Squat
5. Dumbbell/Kettlebell Squat
6. Dumbbell/Kettlebell Pause Squat

Transition to the Barbell Front Rack position

7. Frankenstein Front Squats
8. Lifting Strap Front Squat

At this point, most baseball players may need additional wrist flexibility exercises. A simple exercise to add between Front Squat sets is the **Bench Wrist Stretch.** Do this by rotating your hands so your fingers are facing you and place them on a bench. Do the exercise for 3 sets for 30–45 seconds. You can do this exercise anytime, but you will find it programmed in the Post-Season I (Late Spring/Early Summer) program as we build the Front Squat.

Some baseball players may never fully progress past a front squat with lifting straps and that is fine, provided your program does not include the hang clean.

9. Barbell Front Box Squat
10. Barbell Front Squat

Advancing from the Barbell Front Squat

This is where I introduce the barbell back squat. I have found an athlete is able to learn the barbell back squat much quicker once they have mastered the front squat. I cannot say the opposite is true.

- Barbell Front Pause Squat

- Barbell Back Box Squat

- Barbell Back Squat

- Yoke Bar Squat

- Barbell Back Squat (with chains or bands)

DUMBBELL BENCH PRESS

The bench press is one of the most widely and hotly debated exercises in the world of training baseball players, specifically pitchers. Despite your fears, general upper body strength is essential, especially for high school aged athletes, which is why I prefer dumbbells and push-ups. With dumbbells and push-ups, athletes get a better range-of-motion (a barbell cannot go through your body), a safer range of motion (the head of humerus in not locked into internal rotation), a happy and freely moving scapula, and increased core activation during all single arm bench press and push up variations.

Progression #1	Progression #2	Progression #3	Foundation Movements	Advancement #1	Advancement #2	Advancement #3
Floor Push-Up series	Suspension Trainer Push-Up and/or Dips	Single Arm Dumbbell Bench Press	**Dumbbell Bench Press**	Swiss Barbell (Neutral Grip) Bench Press	Swiss Barbell (Neutral Grip) Close Grip Bench Press	Swiss Barbell (Neutral Grip) Bench Press with Bands or Chains

Building to the Dumbbell Bench Press

1. Hands Elevated Push-Up
2. TRX or Rings Push-Up (45-degree angle) – hands on the handles
3. Floor Push-Up
4. Tempo Push-Up (3 seconds down, pause at the floor, explode up)
5. Feet Elevated Push-Up
6. Floor Pause Push-Up
7. Hand Release Push-Up
8. TRX or Rings Push-Up (parallel to the floor)
9. Dips
10. TRX or Ring Dips
11. Weighted Push-Ups (with a weight vest or lifting chains)
12. Single Arm Dumbbell Bench Press
13. Single Arm Standing Cable Press

Advancing from the Dumbbell Bench Press

1. Swiss Barbell (Neutral Grip) Pause Bench Press
2. Swiss Barbell (Neutral Grip) Close Grip Bench Press
3. Dumbbell or Swiss Barbell (Neutral Grip) Incline Bench Press
4. Swiss Barbell (Neutral Grip) Bench Press with Bands or Chains

But what about the traditional barbell? It comes down to risk versus benefit. A traditional barbell puts your hands in a fixed, pronated (palms down), and slightly internally rotated position which can create undue stress at the shoulder and elbow. In addition, high school boys also tend to turn the barbell into an "ego" lift by loading up too much weight, use horrible technique, and end up setting themselves up for injury, not success. The barbell bench press is not a bad exercise, but it's all in the execution.

For these reasons, I prefer dumbbells and push-ups for the safety and variations they allow.

COACHING POINT

When building to the dumbbell bench press, some larger players will need to be programmed differently than shown above. A player moving 225–275 pounds of bodyweight during a push-up is more a max effort exercise when compared to your 165-pound short stop pumping out 25 reps as a warm-up. Athletes push 60–70 percent of their body weight during a push-up. Therefore, your 250-pound first baseman is pushing 150–175 pounds during each rep. However, you would never load up the bench press with that much weight without a proper warm-up, or for an athlete new to the program. It is fine to push your bigger players towards body weight competency (hands elevated push-ups or rings push-ups) before they "earn" the dumbbells or barbell—just keep in mind the effect of added intensity.

PULL-UP/CHIN-UP

The pull-up (or chin-up) is a versatile movement, easy to add in-between any and all bench and shoulder press sets. This is a great exercise for young, driven student athletes, as it represents the almost primal nature of dominating your own body weight. It also has a direct carryover to your relative strength. Despite this, the pull-up is slowly disappearing from most standard physical education programs.

The pull-up has any number of variations, allowing you to customize to fit your needs, and can even be used as an indicator of an athlete's speed on the field. For example, male players who cannot do a single chin-up are either overweight, weak, or both.

The Pull-up and Chin-up have the added, baseball-specific benefit of training the scapula (shoulder blades). (Scapula strength is also covered in the "Shoulder and Arm Care" section on page 106.) A healthy scapula is allowed freedom of movement north and south (elevation and depression), and east and west (protraction and retraction). A proper Pull-up/Chin-up allows for all four movements and is an amazing exercise to train scapula stability. (See the section on "Mobility vs. Stability" on page 110 for more information).

Progres-sion #1	Progres-sion #2	Progres-sion #3	Foundation Movements	Advance-ment #1	Advance-ment #2	Advance-ment #3
Suspension Trainer Row	Pull-Up/ Chin-Up ISO Holds	Jumping Pull-Up/ Chin-Up NEGATIVES	**Pull-Up/ Chin-Up**	Suspension Trainer Pull-Up	Weighted Pull-Up/ Chin-Up	Multi-Grip Pull-Up/ Chin-Up Mechanical Drop Set

Building to the Pull-Up/Chin-Up

The following progression path makes it easy to build athletes up to the point of being able to confidently execute a Pull-Up correctly.

1. **TRX or Ring Row**
2. **TRX or Ring Row with elevated feet on a box or bench**
3. **Barbell Inverted Row**
4. **Barbell Inverted Row with elevated feet on a box or bench**
5. **Pulldown Machine (work up to 75% body weight)**
6. **Flex Arm Hang**
7. **Pull-up Scapula Retraction and Protraction**
   - From the hang position, pull your shoulder blades down and back. Then allow the shoulder blades to fully retract by relaxing your shoulder blades.
8. **Partner Chin-Up or Pull-Up**
9. **Band Assist Pull-up**
   - Loop a strength band horizontally across a power rack on the "J" cups used for Bench Press and Squat. Choose a height and band resistance that allows you to complete the designated reps. Alternately, loop a band around the pull-up bar so it hangs vertically, then place your foot or knee in the bottom loop.
10. **Chin-Up 5-second Negatives**
    - Use a short box to get your chin above the bar.

11. **Jumping Chin-Up or Pull-Up with a 3 second ISO Hold**
    - Jump from the ground and use that momentum to pull your chin over the bar.

12. **Pull-Up 5-second Negatives.**
    - These are traditional pull-ups with an emphasized negative.

13. **Pull-Up/Chin-Up**

Advancing from the Pull-Up/Chin-Up

When my players can do multiple sets of 12–15 strict reps, I advance them to using a few brutal variations.

- Rotating handles (on a suspension trainer)

- Wide Grip Pull-ups

- Towel Pull-ups (see Forearm Strength on page 105)

- Pause Pull-ups (pausing 2–5 seconds with your chin over the bar at the top of each rep)

- Additional weight (weight vest or lifting chain)

- Intensity techniques (mechanical drop sets – alternate set of Pull-ups and Ring Rows)

COACHING POINT

Even more than with the bench press, it is imperative for the chin-up or pull-up to be programmed differently for your bigger players. When your taller and heavier players use the ring row and pulldown machine, keep in mind the added intensity from their heavier weight.

LUNGE

The majority of sports movements are performed on one leg, which is what makes lunge movements so valuable to every athlete. Lunging improves strength and the ability to change directions while accelerating, decreases injury potential by building side-to-side symmetry, and works to develop stabilizers and balance in a way bilateral exercises (like squats and deadlifts) cannot. Lunges (and their variations) are one of the quickest ways for baseball players to increase their overall athleticism.

In this program, we use the Bulgarian squat as the foundational movement. We do so for a few reasons:

- Most athletes can load a heavy weight in the Bulgarian squat in a matter of months, maybe weeks.

- Barbell walking lunges are simply not feasible in most facilities.

- The elevated rear foot provides more hip mobility than the traditional lunge, which is sorely needed for a generation of players who sit in class all day long.

Progression #1	Progression #2	Progression #3	Foundation Movements	Advancement #1	Advancement #2	Advancement #3
Body Weight Split Squat	Dumbbell Goblet Reverse Lunge	Single Leg Squat (standing on a bench or box)	**Lunge** (Dumbbell Goblet Bulgarian Squat)	Dumbbell Lateral Lunge	Dumbbell Skater Squat	Barbell Reverse or Walking Lunge

Building to the Dumbbell Goblet Bulgarian Squat (Lunge)

- Body Weight Split Squat

- Body Weight Reverse Lunge

- Dumbbell Goblet Reverse Lunge

- Single Leg Squat
  - Stand on a bench or box and heel tap the floor with your balance leg.

- Dumbbell Walking Lunge

Advancing from the Dumbbell Goblet Bulgarian Squat

- Dumbbell Bulgarian Squat
  - Holding two dumbbells at your side allows for more weight.

- Dumbbell Skater Squat
  - Hold two light dumbbells in front of your body for balance. Start the movement similar to a Reverse Lunge, but only allow the back knee to touch the floor.

- Dumbbell 4-Way Lunge (Forward, Reverse, Lateral, Step Behind)

- Barbell Reverse Lunge

- Barbell Forward Lunge

Note that you do not see the barbell Bulgarian squat here. I think the risk outweighs the benefits in a large group setting, with greater potential for balance issues when using the barbell on an athlete's back. If you lose your balance holding a dumbbell, you have a much greater chance to catch yourself. Of course, if you have a small group of good athletes you trust, the barbell Bulgarian squat can be a fine exercise.

Lateral Lunge Variations

The lunge is probably the most multi-faceted exercise offering the most versatility. The lateral lunge and its variations are very important for building lateral glute strength, which can help with quicker first steps, stronger changes of direction, and groin strength.

- Stationary Lateral Lunge

- Pause Stationary Lateral Lunge

- Pause Overhead Stationary Lateral Lunge

- Lateral Squat

- Lateral Sled Walk

- Lateral Lunge

- Cross Over Sled Walk

- Overhead Lateral Lunge

- Pause Lateral Lunge

- Cossack Squat

- 4-Way Lunge (Forward, Reverse, Lateral, Step Behind)

- Pause Overhead Lateral Lunge

COACHING POINT

The slideboard can be an amazing tool for developing lateral deceleration and strength, while building groin (adductor) strength in a non-impact environment. It is also a fantastic tool to condition you laterally. However, I did not program any slideboard workouts for this book because the cost is prohibitive for most athletes and schools. Most go for about $600, and traditionally you will only see slideboards in high-level private facilities, or on college and professional teams.

NEXT LEVEL LUNGES

What if I told you there may be a magical exercise for health, better movement, injury prevention, and sports performance? Enter the Lunge. Hear me out—or better yet, check out these 15 examples and tell me what I missed. Many of these lunges are programmed in the workouts of this book. This section is just as much for my parents and coaches as my athletes. I need my parents and coaches to stay fit and healthy as well!

The Lunge, in all its beautiful variations, checks off a lot of boxes in your pursuit of health, strength, injury prevention, and staying or getting lean.

Cranky knees from 20+ years of Barbell Squat? Try the **Dumbbell Goblet Reverse Lunge.** By stepping backwards into a lunge position, the Reverse Lunge alleviates knee pain by reducing the amount of shear forces on the knee. It also is easier to keep the knee behind your toes, further reducing the shearing force on the knee.

Still love the barbell, but cannot tolerate the Heavy Squat anymore? Try the **Barbell Front Racked Split Squat or Reverse Lunge.** Moving to a single leg squat variation, you are able to lessen the stress on the knee by keeping a more vertical shin, using less total weight, and building the glutes.

Lower back pain? Try the **Walking Lunge with Rotation.** Many times, lower back pain is linked to tight hips. With every step forward, you will feel an amazing stretch in the hip of the back leg. Add in the rotation, and now you have additional thoracic mobility, which is key in alleviating lower back pain.

Tired of cardio but still trying to get leaner? Try **Walking Lunges for Distance.** Ever do Walking Lunges for 1 lap (400 meters) of a track? I did, and I was sore to the touch for five days. Lesson learned. However, going far beyond the traditional 3 sets of 15 reps burns a crazy amount of calories, gets the heart pumping, and even tests your mental fortitude.

Need to get stronger lateral movement or quicker cuts as an athlete? Try **Lateral Lunges.** Athletes in all sports need the ability to move laterally, whether it is staying in front of a defender in basketball, moving along the baseline in tennis, or driving off your back leg to deliver an 85 mph fastball in baseball.

Need more Basic Single Leg Strength? Try the **Split Squat.** Split Squat is a perfect beginner lunge variation.

Need a progression from the Split Squat or more hip mobility? Try the **Front Foot Elevated Split Squat.** Elevate the front foot on a box or bumper plate, 4–8 inches off the ground. The increased range of motion helps build hip mobility.

Want to be sore for three days afterwards? Try the **Bulgarian Squat.** This is also called a Rear Foot Elevated Split Squat. Elevate the back foot on a bench or box, 12–16 inches off the ground. The increased range of motion activates more glutes.

More core and shoulder stability? Try the **Kettlebell Overhead Walking Lunge.** Holding two kettlebells overhead in any position creates the need for more shoulder stability. Add on top of that the walking lunge and now we have a great combination of core stability (keeping an upright position) and shoulder stability (keeping the kettlebells in a locked out position above your head).

More athleticism and power? **Lunge Cycle Jumps.** In addition to lateral movement, every athlete needs more vertical power. Start in a split squat position, jump and switch (cycle) your feet in the air, landing in a lunge position.

More three-dimensional hip mobility? **Lateral Lunge with an Over-head Rotation Reach.** To do this move, lunge to your left while grabbing your left foot with your left hand. While holding the down position of the lateral lunge, reach with your right hand overhead and perform a big, sweeping arm circle. Alternate reps.

Think you're strong? Try the **Skater Squat.** Maybe you can squat three or four plates per side, but I have never seen an exercise humble more "strong" people. Squat down on one leg while lowering the opposite knee (the balance leg will look like a leg curl) to the ground. Lightly tap the opposite knee to the floor (or pad) and stand back up.

Tight hips from sitting at a desk in an office or classroom all day? Try my **3-Way Slider Lunges.** Having tight hips is a multidirectional issue, so it requires a multidirectional answer. To perform 3-Way Slider Lunges, all you need is one furniture slider. You probably have one sitting in your junk drawer right now! This combines three lunge variations as a circuit: Reverse Lunges, Curtsy or Bowler Lunges, and Lateral Lunges.

Returning from a knee injury? Try **Tempo Split Squats.** Most Physical Therapists program tempo work to help rebuild your tendons. Tempo work speaks to an extended repetition. A traditional rep for the purposes of building squat strength is taking 3 seconds to lower the bar, no pause at the bottom, and 1 second (explosively) to squat up. For Tempo Split Squats, take 10 seconds to lower yourself during the squat, no pause at the bottom, and 10 more seconds to stand up. Yes, that is correct, and not a typo. 10 seconds up, 10 seconds down. These brutal sets test your patience, yet are very effective.

Want to emphasize your glute muscles? Try the **Forward Lean Split Squat or Bulgarian Squat.** Adding a slight forward lean to a traditional Split Squat or Bulgarian Squat activates more glutes. You will thank me in the morning!

So, do you believe in magic now? It is hard to argue with the versatility of the lunge!

TIER 2 CORE LIFTS

The next five core lifts are considered Tier 2. These are the movements that truly develop athleticism and a well-rounded athlete. Elements of each are found in every workout, regardless of season or the athlete's level of development. In this section, we'll look at some quick examples of progression for each of these lifts:

1. Jump
2. Carry
3. Rotate and Throw
4. Sprint
5. Core Stability

These five movements (and their variations) are programmed into each workout because they train multi-directional movement, build change of direction strength and speed, and develop general athleticism. See the Progression/Advancement of the Tier 2 Core Lifts section of the table on page 65 for an overview.

HOW TO USE THIS SECTION

In the following pages, we'll discuss in greater detail the types of movements featured in the workout programs of this book and how they relate to the five Tier 2 lift categories listed above. The discussion of each category will feature:

1. An explanation of the role each movement category plays in enhancing an athlete's core fitness.

2. A list of variation exercises for each movement category, for reference. Athletes, especially developing student athletes, thrive on meeting new challenges. By providing a list of different possible exercises that fit in each category, athletes are better able to add variety and personalize their workouts. Certain variations may include additional explanations or step-by-step guides, depending on their general level of difficulty.

3. Coaching points and helpful tips to allow athletes to feel confident as they master the basic movement and progress to its more difficult variations.

Tier 2 Core Lifts in the Workouts

These exercises truly build athleticism. They include all the foundational human movements that athletes need to translate the strength built with the Tier 1 Core Lifts into lasting gains. Generally, the freshman and JV foundation program and the varsity post-season program include progression exercises #1, #2, and #3 (exercises to the left of the foundation movements in the table on page 65), while the advanced exercises (to the right of the foundation movements) are utilized in the varsity in-season, off-season, and pre-season programs.

JUMP

This is the heart of athleticism. Jump training builds the foundation for vertical and horizontal jumps, movement, deceleration, acceleration, and change of direction. Developing the ability to absorb force or decelerate is of the greatest importance for a younger athlete, as that motion always precedes an athlete accelerating or moving in another direction. Your ability to correctly land on a single leg (especially for girls) also directly relates to the long-term health of your knees and prevents ACL tears.

Jump work, also known as **plyometrics,** will typically be found early in a workout, or else will be paired with a strength exercise for the older, varsity athletes in what is called **post-activation potentiation (PAP).** For a full list of drills, see Appendix B: Vertical Jump Playbook on GetFitNow.com.

Progression #1	Progression #2	Progression #3	Foundation Movements	Advancement #1	Advancement #2	Advancement #3
Drop Squat	Drop Split Squat	Depth Drop (off box)	**Jump** (Squat Jump/Broad Jump)	Weighted Squat Jump/ Broad Jump	Depth Drop Squat Jump	Continuous Hurdle Jumps

Jump Progression

A final word on verbiage. I see a lot of confusion regarding jumps vs. bounds vs. hops. Here is your cheat sheet:

• **JUMPS:** Taking off and landing on two legs

• **BOUNDS:** Single leg jumps, landing on the OPPOSITE leg

• **HOPS:** Single leg jumps, landing on the SAME leg

An athlete must be able to decelerate (land) properly before they can accelerate (take off). With that in mind, follow this progression path when building a jump foundation.

First and foremost, you must build towards a proper landing position. Some athletes can achieve this position naturally, by cueing them to get into a "ground ball position." The most efficient and safest landing position always check a few boxes:

• Quarter squat depth (equal parts knee and hip flexion)

• Chest up (be sure you can see the logo on your shirt) with a slight arch in the low back

• Knees are out, over the outside three toes (not leaning/valgus)

- Foot position (width) is based on the athlete's natural landing position

- Neutral head/neck position with the eyes straight ahead

An athlete must be able to establish and hold this position before starting any jump training.

Building to Decelerating/ Absorbing Force Jumps

All "drop" exercises start in a standing position on your toes and then drop into the position listed. Some coaches also refer to these exercise as "snapdowns."

Decelerate/Absorb Force Jumps

- Drop Squat

- Drop Split Squat

- Drop Single Leg Squat
  - Double Leg Standing to Single Leg Squat landing
  - Single Leg Standing to Single Leg Squat landing

- Double Leg Depth Drop (from a box)

- Single Leg Depth Drop (from a box)

Accelerate/Produce Force Jumps

- Squat Jump (Vertical Power)

- Broad Jump (Horizontal Power)

- Lateral Ice Skater Jumps

- Rotational Squat Jumps

- Single Leg Rotational Squat Jump (Jump in place while rotating 90 degrees in either direction)

- Single Leg Rotational Bound (Jump for some distance to the other leg while rotating 90 degrees in either direction)

Hybrid Jumps

These types of jumps combine deceleration and acceleration jumps, e.g. combination of a single leg jump to double leg landings (simple), combination of a double leg jump to a single leg landing (complex). Finally, combine multiple planes of motion—vertical jump to broad jump (vertical to horizontal) or broad jump to lateral broad jump (horizontal to lateral).

- Squat Jump to Broad Jump

- Single Leg Broad Jump to Double Leg Landing

- Single Leg Squat Jump to Double Leg Landing

- Lateral Broad Jump to Squat Jump

- Depth Drop to Broad Jump

- Single Leg Lateral Hop to Forward Sprint

- Single Leg Broad Jump to Squat Jump

To progress most jumps, you can add a weight vest or attach a strength band or bungee for added resistance. Alternatively, add multiple response reps, e.g. multiple squat jumps or broad jumps in a row.

Coaches, if you see any athlete, especially a girl, let their knee fall in (**valgus**) on the jump and/or the landing, add a light mini band around their knees to cue the athletes to activate the glutes and keep the knees in a good athletic position. **Bottom line:** Jump, bound, and hop in all directions to become athletic and explosive!

CARRY

The carry is a self-limiting exercise, one that trains grip strength, core stability, and full body strength all at once. By creating full body tension, it also works to develop mental strength and endurance. To progress the carry, add weight to the movement. All baseball players should build toward the strength to carry dumbbells or trap bar equal to your body weight for 30 yards.

Progres-sion #1	Progres-sion #2	Progres-sion #3	Foundation Movements	Advance-ment #1	Advance-ment #2	Advance-ment #3
Single Arm Overhead Farmer Walk	Single Arm Front Rack Farmer Walk	Single Arm Farmer Walk	**Carry** (Farmer Walk)	Cross Body Farmer Carry	Heavy Trap Bar Farmer Walk	Heavy Trap Bar Single Arm Farmer Walk

Carry Variations

- Farmer Walk (holding dumbbells at each side)

- Single Arm Farmer Walk

- Single Arm Front Rack Farmer Walk

- Single Arm Overhead Farmer Walk

- Cross Body Farmer Carry

- Trap Bar Farmer Walk

- Single Arm Trap Bar (held on your side) Farmer Walk

ROTATE AND THROW

In a book aimed at training baseball players, rotational exercises could easily be considered a Tier 1 exercise, as rotational strength and power are obviously essential for all baseball players. Rotation and throwing exercises go hand in hand; in fact, most medicine ball exercises accomplish both.

Rotation-based exercises push athletes outside of the traditional sagittal plane of movement used by exercises like squats, deadlifts, and bench presses and develops all three planes of movement—the sagittal, the frontal and the transverse—to create better athleticism and greater force transfer. Throw exercises are done by jumping up and down, forwards and backwards with a medicine ball, and therefore have a direct carry-over effect on your athleticism.

To progress rotation and throw exercises, use heavier weights (like a heavier medicine ball) or look to throw for further distance or with greater speed. You can also try adding a hop or jump before the throw. Finally, add weight or speed to the movement to progress cable- or band-based rotation exercises.

Progres-sion #1	Progres-sion #2	Progres-sion #3	Foundation Movements	Advance-ment #1	Advance-ment #2	Advance-ment #3
Cable Lift	Cable Chop	Cable Pallof Press	**Rotate** (Cable Rotation)	Lunge Cable Lift/ Chop/ Pallof Press	Medicine Ball Rotation Throw	Medicine Ball Lateral Hop Rotation Throw
Medicine Ball Scoop Throw	Medicine Ball Reverse Scoop Throw	Medicine Ball Acceleration Throw	**Throw** (Medicine Ball Squat Press Throw)	Medicine Ball Rapid Response Overhead Throw	Medicine Ball Rapid Response Linear Throw	Medicine Ball Rapid Response Lateral Throw

Rotate Variations

- Rotational Medicine Ball Throws (for distance)
- Rotational Medicine Ball Throws (catch and throw off the wall)
  - Facing the wall and standing perpendicular to the wall
  - Kneeing, Half-Kneeling, Lunge, or Standing positions
- Lateral Bound Rotational Medicine Ball Throws
- Machine Cable or Band Exercises
  - Cable Rotations
  - Cable Paloff Press
  - Cable Chop
  - Cable Lift

Throw Variations

- Medicine Ball Squat Press Throw
- Medicine Ball Reverse Scoop Throw
- Medicine Ball Acceleration Throw

SPRINT

Since the game of baseball revolves around repeated, short, maximum-intensity bursts of jumps and sprints, the ability to generate force, change direction, and rapidly decelerate tends to be the determining factor between reaching that ball in the hole or not, or beating out that ground ball for a hit. Therefore, a holistic sprint (speed) program must include elements of acceleration and deceleration, lateral movement, change of direction, and reactive agility to be worthwhile for a baseball player.

This section is less of a progression path than a combination of drills to increase your movement speed. After all, it is a little difficult to teach running technique from reading words on a page! For a full list of drills, see Appendix A: Speed Development Playbook on GetFitNow.com.

Progres- sion #1	Progres- sion #2	Progres- sion #3	Foundation Movements	Advance- ment #1	Advance- ment #2	Advance- ment #3
Wall drills and dynamic warm up for technique	Plyometric jumps for power and acceleration	Sled push for resisted speed and acceleration	**Sprint**	Change of Direction/ Speed	Reaction Agility Speed	Over Speed Training

Sprint Variations

Deceleration

- Banded or Bungee Lateral Walk

- Banded or Bungee Lateral Shuffle

Acceleration

- Light Sled Push

- Hill Sprints

- Stadium Stairs

- 10-yard Chase Sprint

Change of Direction

- 3 Cone Drill
- 60-yard Shuttle Run
- Pro Agility (5-10-5 Drill)
- "W" Drill
- "T" Drill

Reactive Agility (Cognitive)

- Push-Up Sprints
- 20-yard sprints, starting on code word trigger (like "RED")

Reactive Agility (Visual)

- Competition Push-Up Sprints
- 20-yard sprints, starting on first movement of lead athlete

Reactive Agility (Verbal)

- Competition Half Kneeling Sprints
- 20-yard sprints, starting on verbal instruction (like "GO")

Over Speed

- Light Assist Sprint (Band, Bungee, or Tow Strap)
- Downhill (last 5-10 feet) Sprint

Full Speed

- Swim Noodle Chase Drill

CORE STABILITY

Core stability must be a focus of all high school athletes. Most kids sit 6–8 hours of the day in class, developing tight hips and poor posture as a result. Then we ask them to squat, deadlift, and be athletic—without addressing their core stability—and wonder why they develop back pain! An emphasis on core stability will help prevent back pain in young baseball players still growing into his or her body.

However, what is the difference between core stability and core strength?

Core stability is the capacity to reduce, produce, and stabilize force through the trunk/torso area while maintaining a neutral lumbar spine (such as is used during overhead squats and deadlifts). This is the primary purpose of your core and will keep you strong and injury-free in the long run. The primary function of your "core" is not all those crunches you have been doing, but my five core stability groups:

- Anterior core stability (anti-extension)

- Posterior core stability (anti-flexion)

- Lateral core stability (anti-lateral flexion)

- Rotary core stability (anti-rotation)

- Hip flexion with neutral spine

Core strength is the body's capacity to flex, extend, bend and rotate the spine, using your core muscles as the primary movers. Focusing on core strength is the old-school way of training your core, using exercises like crunches, sit-ups, back hyperextensions and side bends, as well as rotational exercises like the Russian twist (which research shows is terrible for your lower back).

So, if focusing on core strength is the old-fashioned way of doing things, does this mean you should never crunch again?

The answer is, of course not. However, it does mean that crunches should not be your primary method of training your core muscles. Leading low back researcher Shirley Sahrmann wrote:

"During most daily activities, the primary role of the abdominal muscles is to provide isometric support and limit the degree of rotation of the trunk…A large percentage of low back problems occur because the abdominal muscles are not maintaining tight control over the rotation between the pelvis and the spine at the L5–S1 level."

Further, physical therapists Porterfield and DeRosa stated, "Rather than considering the abdominals as flexors and rotators of the trunk–for which they certainly have the capacity–their function might be better viewed as anti-rotators and anti-lateral flexors of the trunk."

Progression #1	Progression #2	Progression #3	Foundation Movements	Advancement #1	Advancement #2	Advancement #3
Core Stability PREP Program	Dead Bug Variations	Physioball Plank Circles	**Core Stability** Suspension Trainer Plank Rollouts	Ab Wheel Kneeling Rollouts	Single Arm Front Plank variations	Ab Wheel Pushup Rollouts

COACHING POINT

It is very important to build the core stability of athletes, especially taller and younger players, to prevent future issues with soft tissue lower back strains. You should be dedicating at least 5–10 minutes of each in-season lift to direct core stability workouts. The goal is to keep athletes fresh, healthy, and ready to come back for the next game. This can have a profound effect on the lower back health of taller and younger players who simply don't have the core stability needed to compete at the varsity level.

FRESHMAN AND JV CORE STABILITY PROGRAM

The following core stability prep program is built into the freshman and JV foundation workouts found in this book, as well as the varsity GPP workouts in the post-season winter months. This core stability program keeps players out of the athletic training room and the head coach happy.

Core Stability PREP Program

Exercise	Sets	Reps/Time	You Pass If...
Plank	4	60 seconds	Can hold a neutral spine and feel the core muscle fire for the entire 60 seconds
Side Plank	4	45 seconds per side	Can hold a neutral spine with your top shoulder, back, and hips up for the entire 45 seconds, each side
Alternate Leg Raise	4	12 each leg	Can heel tap the floor with one foot while creating a 90-degree angle between your legs and keeping your lower back FLAT to the floor
Back Extension ISO (holds)	4	60 seconds	Can hold a neutral spine and keep your glutes contracted with your hands on your head for the entire 60 seconds

Core Stability Progressions

Anterior core stability (anti-extension)

- Physioball Plank Circles

- Suspension Trainer Plank Rollouts

- Ab Wheel Kneeling Rollouts

- Ab Wheel Pushup Rollouts

Posterior core stability (anti-flexion)

- Floor Back Extension

- 45-degree Bench Back Extension

- Glute Ham Bench Back Extension

- Barbell Good Morning

Lateral core stability (anti-lateral flexion)

- Side Plank + Top Knee Drive (pull the top knee into your chest each rep)

- Side Plank + Top Leg Raise (raise your top leg 6–12" reach rep)

- Side Plank + Inside Knee Drive (pull the bottom knee into your chest each rep)

- Single Arm Farmer Carry

Rotary core stability (anti-rotation)

- Dead Bug Variations

- Single Arm Front Plank variations

- Dumbbell Renegade Row

- Pallof Press

- Landmine Rotations

- Dumbbell Bird Dog Row

- All single arm and single leg dumbbell exercises

Hip flexion with neutral spine

- Floor Alternate Leg Drive, Raise, and Circles

- Physioball Alternate Leg Drive, Raise, and Circles

- Physioball or Slider Knee Tucks (Jackknives)

- Hang Knee Raise or Leg Raise

TIER 3 CORE LIFTS

The final five movements are considered Tier 3. These are the movements that fill in the gaps left by the Tier 1 and Tier 2 movements. These movements (and their variations) are programmed into most workouts because they train hip extension (crucial in vertical jump and speed development), strengthen the muscles surrounding the knee, and provide balance to your upper body training. In this section, we'll look at some quick examples of progression for each of these lifts:

1. Glute Bridge (Hip Extension)
2. Leg Curl (Knee Flexion)
3. Leg Extension (Backward Sled Pull)
4. Shoulder Press (Vertical Push)
5. Row (Horizontal Row)

See the Progression/Advancement of the Tier 3 Core Lifts section of the table on page 66 for an overview.

HOW TO USE THIS SECTION

In the following pages, we'll discuss in greater detail the types of movements considered Tier 3 for the purposes of the workout programs in this book.

The discussion of each category will feature:

1. An explanation of the role each movement category plays in enhancing an athlete's core fitness.
2. A list of variation exercises for each movement category, for reference. These variations provide student athletes with the opportunity to explore each movement category and select the specific exercises that work best for their fitness goals.

Tier 3 Core Lifts in the Workouts

Each of these exercises fills a specific gap left in your physical development by the Tier 1 and 2 Core Lifts. The glute bridge exercises, for example, build hip extension (more speed and explosive jumps) without additional stress to the lower back and support healthy knees, while the leg curl exercises strengthen the hamstring at the knee and balance out hamstring development.

While these movements would greatly benefit freshman and JV players, there is simply not enough training time in a typical workout that focuses on Tier 1 and 2 exercises to include most of the Tier 3 exercises. Tier 3 exercise are less a progression, and more a list of exercise variations (assistance exercises) for the varsity player, to be used in the off-season and pre-season programs.

GLUTE BRIDGE (HIP EXTENSION)

While the deadlift, squat, and lunge activate the glutes, the glute bridge (and its variations) destroy the glutes without creating an additional load on the lower back. This is especially important with today's athletes, where the glutes tend to be underactive and lead to tight hips. This can create an environment of lower back pain and weak core stability and strength. Also, stronger glutes leads to greater speed and explosion!

Progres-sion #1	Progres-sion #2	Progres-sion #3	Foundation Movements	Advance-ment #1	Advance-ment #2	Advance-ment #3
Glute Bridge	Single Leg Glute Bridge	Single Leg Hip Thrust	**Barbell Glute Bridge**	Barbell Hip Thrust	Kettlebell Single Leg Hip Thrust	3D Barbell Hip Thrust

Glute Bridge Variations

- Glute Bridge

- Single Leg Glute Bridge

- Glute Bridge (feet elevated on box or bench)

- Single Leg Glute Bridge (feet elevated on box or bench)

- Single Leg Hip Thrust

- Kettlebell Single Leg Hip Thrust

- Banded Hip Thrust

- Banded Single Leg Hip Thrust

- Barbell Glute Bridge

- Barbell Hip Thrust

- 3D Barbell Hip Thrust (Sling Shot around knees)

- Barbell Hip Thrust with Chains or Band resistance

Glute Bridge vs Hip Thrust

You may be wondering, "What is the difference?" Simple: Both are hip extension movements, but the Glute Bridge works with your shoulders on the floor and the Hip Thrust works with the shoulder elevated on a box or bench. The Hip Thrust is a progression because of the added range of motion and because it activates more quad and glute muscles.

LEG CURL (KNEE FLEXION)

While the deadlift, squat, and lunge activate the hamstrings, they do so primarily at the hip. For complete hamstring development and knee stability, you must have exercises that strengthen the hamstring at the knees as well.

Progres-sion #1	Progres-sion #2	Progres-sion #3	Foundation Movements	Advance-ment #1	Advance-ment #2	Advance-ment #3
Physioball Glute Bridge	Physioball Leg Curl	Physioball Single Leg Curl	**Slider Leg Curl**	Slider Single Leg Curl	Glute Ham Raise	Nordic/ Russian Leg Curl

Leg Curl Variations

- Machine (Prone or Seated) Leg Curl

- Machine (Prone or Seated) Single Leg Curl

- Physioball Leg Curl

- Physioball Single Leg Curl

- Slider Leg Curl Negatives

- Slider Leg Curl

- Slider Single Leg Curl Negatives

- Slider Single Leg Curl

- Glute Ham Raise

- Nordic/Russian Leg Curl

LEG EXTENSION (BACKWARD SLED PULL)

While squats and lunges work the quads (especially the front squat and short step lunge variations), leg extension exercises hammer your vastus medialus obliquus (or VMO). Also known as the "teardrop" muscle, the VMO is a key muscle in knee stabilization.

Progression #1	Progression #2	Progression #3	Foundation Movements	Advancement #1	Advancement #2	Advancement #3
Banded Spanish Squat ***Band behind the kneecap	Banded Split Squat ***Band behind the kneecap	Machine Single Leg Extension focused on the last 30 degrees of extension	**Backward Sled Pull**	Backward Sled Pull and Row	Lighter weights for speed and heavier weights for strength	Alternate Backward and Forward Sled Push

Backward Sled Pull Variations

- Banded Spanish Squat

- Banded Split Squat

- Machine Leg Extension

- Machine Single Leg Extension

- Backward Sled Pull

- Backward Sled Pull and Row

- Light (50% body weight) Backward Sled Pull (for speed)

- Longer distance, moderate (100% body weight) for distance

- Heavy (150% body weight) for strength

- Alternate Backward and Forward Sled Push

SHOULDER PRESS (VERTICAL PUSH)

The shoulder press, or vertical push movement, complements the Tier 1 horizontal push core lift, the bench press. Overhead press is no longer forbidden for baseball players, especially for healthy players with no injury history at the shoulder.

Are *you* ready to Overhead Press? Here's a checklist:

1. Have you mastered Thoracic Spine extension?
2. Do you have good core stability?
3. Are you free from Upper Crossed Syndrome?

If yes to all three, you're good to go!

Any players, pitchers included, who can properly extend in the Thoracic (mid-back) Spine while maintaining good core stability (no excessive extension/arch in the lower back) without Upper Crossed Syndrome (see our section on *Shoulder and Arm Care* on page 106) is a great candidate for the overhead press. Even with all that said, it still comes down to a risk versus benefit analysis, which is why the majority of all my overhead pressing is done with a neutral grip and single arm.

Progression #1	Progression #2	Progression #3	Foundation Movements	Advancement #1	Advancement #2	Advancement #3
½ Kneeling Landmine or Dumbbell Press	Lunge Landmine or Dumbbell Press	Dumbbell Single Arm Shoulder Press	**Dumbbell Shoulder Press**	SWIS Barbell (Neutral Grip) Z Press	SWIS Barbell (Neutral Grip) Shoulder Press	Dumbbell or SWIS Barbell (Neutral Grip) Push Press

Shoulder Press Variations

- ½ Kneeling Landmine Press (back knee on the floor)

- Lunge Landmine Press (back knee off the floor)

- ½ Kneeling Dumbbell Shoulder Press

- ½ Kneeling Single Arm Dumbbell Shoulder Press

- Lunge Dumbbell Shoulder Press

- Lunge Single Arm Dumbbell Shoulder Press

- Dumbbell Single Arm Standing Shoulder Press

- Dumbbell Standing Shoulder Press

- SWIS Barbell Shoulder Press

- Floor (Seated) Dumbbell or SWIS Barbell Shoulder Press (Z Press)

ROW (HORIZONTAL ROW)

The row and its variations complement the Tier 1 vertical pull movement, the pull-up/chin-up. The row is important for high school athletes because it can help restore proper posture after sitting at a desk for 6–8 hours each day. The row also provides muscular balance to even out all the shoulder press and bench pressing in the program to help maintain happy shoulders. (I also include rear deltoid and other shoulder prehab exercises in this category for this reason.)

Progres-sion #1	Progres-sion #2	Progres-sion #3	Foundation Movements	Advance-ment #1	Advance-ment #2	Advance-ment #3
Suspension Trainer Row	Barbell Inverted Row	Dumbbell Supported Row	**Dumbbell One-Arm Row**	Dumbbell Row	Landmine Row	Barbell Row

Row Variations

In a book aimed at training baseball players, row exercises could easily be considered a Tier 1 exercise, as row exercise is essential for shoulder health in all baseball players.

- Band Pull-Aparts

- Band Side External Rotations

- 3–5 lbs. Dumbbell Prone "T" Raise

- Suspension Trainer Row

- Barbell Inverted Row

- Dumbbell Supported Row

- Dumbbell One-Arm Row

- Dumbbell Row

- Landmine Row

- Barbell Row

TRAINING TARGET AREAS

I n addition to the core movements discussed in the previous sections, there are specific target areas and training goals that any baseball athlete should look to improve. These range from building forearm strength, creating shoulder and arm care programs, mobility, force production, speed development, and conditioning.

FOREARM STRENGTH

Strong forearms and baseball go hand and hand. As one of the few muscles actually exposed in a baseball uniform, a yoked-up set of forearms and a killer handshake are what really separate the baseball player from other athletes.

Forearms are predominantly **Type I, slow-twitch muscles fibers,** which means they respond best to high volumes of reps (12–25) per set. However, we still train them using traditional strength protocols (4–8 reps for 3–4 sets) to ensure complete forearm development.

Training the forearm also takes more than curls and extensions. The forearm's range of motion includes **supination and pronation,** or rotating the wrist and the hands, palms up to palms down. Finally, they can also **ulnar and radial deviate the wrist,** which is best described as the movement of the wrist from side to side while moving your thumb towards your forearm (radial) and your little finger towards your forearm (ulnar).

Combine these six movements with a mix of rep schemes and multiple pieces of equipment, and you have the making of a forearm that can turn singles into doubles and doubles into BOMBS!

For a list of all my favorite forearm exercises with six specific programs, see www.GetFitNow.com.

This Forearm Strength Playbook covers the four major areas that build forearm strength:

1. Grip Strength Focus by holding heavy weights (isometrics) in a variety of methods.
2. Forearm Strength focuses on the six forearm movements discussed in the section on page 105.
3. Weighted Bat Drills
4. Forearm Focus Weight Room Exercises

SHOULDER AND ARM CARE

Shoulder care can mean rotator cuff work, jobes, "scap" work, or multi-purpose shoulder programs—but however you choose to do it, taking care of the muscles surrounding a player's throwing shoulder is paramount. During my years in professional baseball as a strength and conditioning coach, this was the biggest point of emphasis for the coordinators during a visit or a weekly call about pitchers. In addition to the higher probability of shoulder injuries from simply playing baseball, high school players today sit hunched at a school desk for 6–8 hours per day, which creates "upper crossed syndrome": poor posture, tight pecs and internally rotated arms, and weak upper back and scapula muscles.

Think of this as a public service announcement to all players: **shoulder care is your responsibility!** The devil is in the details when performing the majority of these exercises; strength coaches and athletic trainers can program and prescribe them, but it is the player who must have the focus, attention to detail, and commitment to do them properly and consistently.

For a list of all my favorite shoulder and arm targeted prehab exercises, with five specific programs, see www.GetFitNow.com.

This Shoulder and Arm Care Playbook covers the five major areas that affect shoulder care:

1. Shoulder mobility
2. Scapula stability
3. Rotator cuff health
4. Thoracic spine mobility
5. Core stability

IMPROVING MOBILITY

For newer athletes, proper mobility drills and warm-ups are the toughest things to learn. Part of this is the terminology involved; everyone knows what a squat or deadlift is, yet with the recent explosion in mobility programs, the number of "trademarked" or "modified" movements, each with their own designation, has many players confused.

Therefore, I wanted to create a short and sweet mobility menu, incorporating the "Big 5" and Olympic movements. These exercises form the foundation of all movement meant to promote strength and balance while reducing the chance for injury. The goal for every baseball player is to have a full range of motion (proper mobility), allowing them to be pain-free, injury-free and perform at their most effective and efficient level.

For over 100 mobility exercises, please check out *The Mobility Workout Handbook: Over 100 Sequences for Improved Performance, Reduced Injury, and Increased Flexibility.*

MOBILITY MENU: THE TOP 10 FOR THE "BIG 5"

Squat and Deadlift Mobility

The emphasis here is on the ankle, hip, and thoracic spine, as well as the core and knee stability.

1. Single Leg Glute Bridge
2. Lunge Yoga Rotations
3. PVC Bench Thoracic Extension
4. Medicine Ball Thoracic Extension
5. Kneeling Thoracic Rotations
6. Floor Medicine Ball Thoracic Rotations
7. Band Overhead Squat Pattern
8. Walking Lunge with Rotation
9. Dumbbell "T" Balance
10. PVC or Barbell Overhead Squat

Bench, Pull-Up, and Shoulder Press Mobility

The emphasis here is on the hip, shoulder and thoracic spine, as well as the core and scapula stability.

1. Yoga Push-Up
2. Band Pull-Aparts
3. PVC Bench Thoracic Extension
4. Medicine Ball Thoracic Extension
5. Kneeling Thoracic Rotations
6. Dumbbell "T" Raise (Rear Delt Raise)
7. Foam Roll Latissimus Dorsi (Lat) Muscles

8. PVC or Barbell Overhead Squat

9. Lunge Yoga Rotations

10. Band Overhead Squat Pattern

Olympic Mobility

The emphasis here is on the ankle, hip, thoracic spine, shoulder and wrist, as well as the core, knee and scapula stability.

1. Bench Wrist Stretch

2. PVC Bench Thoracic Extension

3. Medicine Ball Thoracic Extension

4. Kneeling Thoracic Rotations

5. PVC or Barbell Overhead Squat

6. Foam Roll Latissimus Dorsi (Lat) Muscles

7. ISO Front Squat (hold the bottom of Barbell Front Squat)

8. Wall Half Kneeling 3-Way Ankle Mobility

9. Lunge Yoga Rotations

10. Single Leg Glute Bridge

MOBILITY VS. STABILITY

Football coach Herm Edward is famous for saying, "The best ability is durability." I believe we can take that phrase to the next level: "The best ability is durability; the best durability is **mobility and strength**." An athlete's ability to stay durable—to stay on the field—is their ability to stay mobile and strong.

This opens up a bigger discussion on **mobility vs. stability.**
Mobility is defined as the ability to *produce* a desired movement.
Stability, by contrast, is the ability to *resist* an undesired movement.

Mobility and stability occurs during all the "Big 5" exercises, at multiple joints, with every rep.

Coaches must have a basic understanding on how the human body moves beyond the Squat, Bench, Deadlift, and Clean. Mike Boyle and Gray Cook popularized a framework to help simplify the confusing mobility vs. stability discussion. This joint by joint approach is an outline that tells us, in general terms, if a joint needs to be stable or mobile during play. The basics of their outline is included below:

MOBILE	STABLE
Ankle	Foot
Hip	Knee
Thoracic Spine (T-spine)	Lumbar Spine
Shoulder	Cervical Spine
Wrist	Scapula

Players must spend more time on mobility and stability in areas that were sites of previous injury. Any area that has sustained an injury is more susceptible to re-injury, but diligent mobility and stability work can help. A good piece of advice for all players with an injury history is to perform a shortened version of your last physical therapy workout two or three times per week.

BUILDING FORCE PRODUCTION

Many people believe the primary objective of plyometric exercise is to increase our ability to *produce* force, but in actuality, it serves to help us *absorb* force. Confused? The ability to produce force is limited by your ability to absorb force. You can only change directions or jump in the air *after* you have *absorbed* the opposing force. In addition, the quicker and more efficiently you can decelerate your body, the quicker and more powerfully you will accelerate.

This is called the **stretch shortening cycle.** Deceleration precedes all acceleration. Go ahead, try this right now! Stand up, and jump in the air as high as you can. Did you notice you had to bend your hips, knees, and ankles to jump up? Bending your hips, knees, and ankles was deceleration. Therefore, the greater speed and strength with which you can decelerate, the greater the force you can produce and the height you can jump. You can also move significantly faster if you can stop quicker.

BUILDING DECELERATION IN THE WEIGHT ROOM

Every rep we do in the weight room includes three contractions:

1. Concentric: **produces** force
2. Isometric: **stabilizes** force
3. Eccentric: **reduces** force

For example, the barbell front squat. Eccentric force occurs when you descend (sit down) during the squat. Isometric force is the transfer of energy from down to up. Concentric force occurs when you ascend (stand up) during the squat.

In his book *Triphasic Training*, Carl Dietz dives deeply into all three contractions. Dietz writes: "Every dynamic movement begins with an eccentric muscle action."

Therefore, to build better deceleration and subsequent acceleration and power, you must focus on the eccentric and isometric contractions in the weight room. It goes beyond just performing reps "slow and controlled."

Let's go a bit deeper.

Eccentric Based Training

Dietz suggests using only large, compound exercises (think the "Big 5") with an accentuated (slow) eccentric phase. Traditional strength programs and coaches will program "slow and controlled" reps in the 2–3 seconds range. Dietz's protocols call for a total eccentric time of 5–8 seconds per rep. That can be twice the time you and your athletes are used to being in the eccentric phase. It will feel like an eternity for the first couple of workouts.

Dietz gives four rules to follow for eccentric based training:

1. Only use large, compound exercises (squat, bench, deadlift, and lunges) and go into them early in the workout when the athlete is fresh.
2. Do not exceed 85% of an athlete's 1 rep max.
3. Always, always spot the athlete during slow eccentrics.
4. Always finish each eccentric focused rep with an explosive, concentric movement.

REAL LIFTING AND PHYSICAL THERAPY

Many physical therapists will program **tempo sets** (accentuated eccentric and/or concentric phase) into their rehab programs in order to appropriately load and stress the tendon to stimulate and promote healing and regeneration. Dr. Benjamin Fan of Next Level Physical Therapy says: "Research has found heavy slow resistance (HSR) training to be effective in treating patella tendinopathies (nagging knee pain in the front of the kneecap), finding improvements in not only the short term, but also long term. This involves a person performing a movement (squat, leg press, or hack squat) with a tempo. The tempos can range from 5–10 seconds for all three muscle contractions—eccentric, isometric, and concentric."

You can also program tempo versions of this principle. An example would be:

Tempo Dumbbell Goblet Squat

> 5 seconds eccentric (down)
> 0 seconds isometric (hold)
> 5 seconds concentric (up)

Perform for 6 reps, or 60 seconds. Build up to 3 sets. (It is *so* much harder than it seems on paper!)

Isometric Based Training

Perhaps the most difficult to explain, isometric contractions transfer your eccentric force into explosive concentric force (explosive changes of direction.

Dietz offers a few rules to follow for isometric-based training:

1. Find the joint angle(s) your athletes explode from and focus on training those areas in the weight room. Think of a ground ball position.

2. Only use large, compound exercises (squat, bench, deadlift, and lunges) and go into them early in the workout when the athlete is fresh.

3. "Hit the ground like a brick;" i.e., perform the preceding eccentric motion at full speed to teach your body to absorb 100% of that eccentric force.

4. Master the body weight isometric positions before adding a barbell or dumbbells.

5. Always, always spot the athlete during slow eccentrics.

6. Always finish each isometric focused rep with an explosive concentric movement.

SPEED DEVELOPMENT

An athlete's speed is based on proper stride length, stride frequency and force production into the ground. The game of baseball is primarily composed of repeated, short, maximum-intensity bouts of exercise with extended periods of rest. The ability to generate force, accelerate, change directions, and reach top speed tends to be a separator for athletes. Your speed workouts must therefore focus on these demands by training the basic qualities of speed.

Mechanical Basics of Linear Speed

Keep toes pulled up toward shins. Cue athletes to keep "TOES UP!" to initiate knee and hip flexion quicker.

Drive knees up and avoid over striding. Feet in front of the body = BRAKES; feet behind the body = ACCELERATION; feet underneath the body = max VELOCITY (breakaway speed).

Fire glutes and hamstrings to apply force into ground. This is why we focus on the posterior chain so much in the weight room.

Aggressively drive the elbows forward and back from cheek to cheek. This can account for 5–10 percent of speed potential.

Point chin slightly down, focus eyes straight ahead and hold head still. Maintaining a core upright posture allows the muscles to fire correctly.

Relax upper-body muscles and face. Muscles fire better when relaxed.

Constructing Speed Workouts

The speed workouts in this book are more drill-based than technical-based. Just as you cannot learn how to hit or pitch a baseball from a book, it is even harder to learn proper speed mechanics just by reading about them. Therefore, we have programmed for and included drills that put the athlete in proper athletic positions with minimal technique exercises.

Let us briefly run down the elements of a speed workout, and the function each serves in developing young baseball players. Any speed workout must focus on the physical demands of baseball by training these qualities of speed.

You can also find a database of exercises for each of these speed development categories, as well as a list of uncommon exercises for quick reference at GetFitNow. com/extras.

Dynamic Warm-Ups

The benefits of dynamics have been covered extensively. When programming for dynamic warm-ups, choose movements that mimic that day's work out. Is it a "Lateral Speed and Agility" day? Work on lateral base skips, carioca quick steps, and micro hurdle lateral skips. Acceleration Day? Work acceleration skips, linear agility ladder drills, and micro hurdle linear skips into the mix.

Mobility

This step is perhaps the most often skipped by young athletes. Moving your ankles and hips through a full range of motion for max speed and acceleration is so important, especially as it will help prevent injury and improve flexibility.

Plyometrics

Power production (acceleration and deceleration) is a priority for all athletes, which is why it is best done when athletes are fresh (i.e., early in the workout) and loose (after the warm-up). Multi-directional (linear, lateral, and rotational) jumps and throws are best.

Acceleration

Program for short bursts of 10–20-yard (30-60 feet) drills designed to work on your forward lean while maximizing your force production on the ground. Sled pushes, hill sprints, and stadium stairs are staples.

Change of Direction

For proper athletic development, athletes need to develop the skill of deceleration. An athlete's ability to plant their foot quickly and efficiently is one of the most important athletic qualities they can possess. Short shuttle and run down drills should be the focus here.

Reactive Agility

This training challenges athletes with visual, audio and cognitive cues on your traditional "agility drills." For example, coaches will use the following types of cues:

- **Visual:** Pointing out the direction

- **Audio:** Calling out directions

- **Cognitive:** Calling out a color associated with a particular direction

Drills are also made more effective by performing them from different starting positions, such as lying face down (prone) or lying face up (supine) position. Taken a step further, you can lie face up or face down with your head facing towards the intended sprint or away. My favorite, and most versatile, are lunge starts, as these more closely simulate game situations. Think of the many lunge variations in the Tier 1 section on page 80.

Over Speed

Assisted speed, or over speed training, is best for improving stride length. Again, speed is stride length times stride frequency with max force production into the ground. The key here is to push your limits (add about 5–10% extra) without a breakdown in your running technique. If you force your body to move too fast, your feet will be hitting in front of your body, which correlates to slamming on the brakes, not reaching max velocity. Downhill running (the last 5–10 feet), bungee, and band assisted sprints are best.

Circle Sprints

Some coaches refer to this training as Curvilinear Speed. I prefer simplicity, so circle sprints it is. Circle sprints specifically build base running speed. When doing circle sprints, coaches can manipulate the curve of the circle to accommodate for intensity. The greater (tighter) the curve, the greater the intensity. For example, sprinting around the pitcher's mound is much more difficult than sprinting around the edge of the infield grass. Circle sprint drills are also great for not only body awareness (leaning towards the direction you are sprinting), but for ankle strength (supination/pronation) as well. Running the bases is a very one-sided activity, so using circle drills in both directions to balance the body is very important.

Full Speed

While often overlooked, you do need to sprint in order to get faster. Speed development (as opposed to conditioning, see below) requires full recovery between sets to allow for maximal effort. Full speed drills of 90 feet (single) or 180 feet (doubles) that focus on team competition and full speed chases/races are best.

Cool Down Stretch and Foam Roll Massage

Start the recovery cycle as soon as you are done with your last sprint to prepare your body for tomorrow's lift. Grab a foam roller or tennis ball to massage trigger points in the body to help prepare you for the day's workout. Massaging releases the knots, adhesions, and scar tissue that build up from the trauma of exercise and allow you to increase blood flow and circulation to the soft tissues. Finish summer conditioning workouts with an ice roller (a frozen 2-liter bottle), which offers the benefits of massage and ice all in one!

BASEBALL CONDITIONING

There are a million and one different conditioning tests and drills; long gone are the days of the 1.5-mile test, timing poles, and running for punishment (I hope). So, which test is best?

The answer is, whichever one best suits your needs, your players, and is something that you and your staff can run effectively and efficiently. In addition, it is of the utmost importance that the head baseball coach is on the same page as the strength and conditioning coach when it comes to conditioning. Ultimately, conditioning is not something that requires or reflects baseball talent; however, it does let you know who busted their tail over the winter and fall and is ready for pre-season camp or season play. However, it can allow the talented pitcher to pitch late into games.

That said, designing a new conditioning test is hard work, and something that requires a lot of trial and error. Ideally, conditioning drills should contain work to rest ratios that mimic game situations, incorporate game skills, and follow the desired pace and tempo that coincides with the head coach's philosophy.

The key? **Repeat sprint ability.** The ability to repeat near full speed sprints is paramount in baseball. It is also baseball-specific and matches the energy system used in games (see below). To excel in baseball, players are required to not only produce a great deal of power (jump, swing, throw), but do so repeatedly (sprint).

Finally, well-designed practices can act as the best form of conditioning. It can specifically match what is expected of the players in a game and avoid having the players run separately. Any player knows in their heart of hearts that they give more intensity and effort during all the hard fought competitions and drills in practice than when running extra poles after practice and running separately.

Baseball Energy Systems

There is no "average" baseball game, meaning it is very difficult to quantify a position player's average number of sprints or changes of direction or the number of pitches a pitcher will throw. However, we can all agree on the two levels of intensity during a game:

1. **High:** Outfielder sprinting after a fly ball, infielder sprinting into the hole or up the middle, catcher backing up first base, pitching, and hitting.

2. **Low:** Walking, timeouts, time in between pitches, rests on the bench

We see an average of 25 seconds between pitches, but how many "reps" or plays you see, or pitches and duration spent at each level of intensity, is very position-specific.

- **Pitchers** can take 1–3 seconds to deliver a pitch, meaning an average of 15 pitches per inning. That equates to about 90 pitches for 6 innings and about 105 pitches for 7 innings. Both are considered quality starts.

- **Catchers** are squatting all game and must back up first base on most ground balls.

- **Infielders** accelerate, sprint, and change direction each round and are in constant motion, backing up plays and for pickoffs.

- **Outfielders** sprint to all fly balls and any balls hit into the gaps. The corner outfielders in particular are in constant motion to back up first and third base.

- **Baserunners** have the most variability: sprinting to first, second, and third base, going first to third, second to home, stealing second base, etc.

Now, how does your body deal with this type of irregular energy demand? The primary energy system utilized by the body during baseball is **anaerobic,** while the secondary energy system is **aerobic capacity.** The anaerobic energy system of the body is quick, explosive, and is used for full speed sprints, pitching, hitting, and jumps lasting less than 10 seconds and which are followed by a brief rest or of lesser intensity. (Sound familiar? That is the game of baseball!) Aerobic capacity refers to an athlete's ability to recover quickly between plays, recovery day to day and between double headers. You can test your aerobic capacity by taking your rest heart rate. A well-conditioned baseball player should have less than 60 beats per minute.

If you're at over 60 beats per minute, realize that your resting heart rate can fluctuate daily, and a high number may just indicate that you have yet to recover from yesterday's hard practice or game. Therefore, you should take your pulse each morning for 3–5 days in a row to get a baseline.

Combining these two energy systems should be the bedrock of any conditioning program, especially for the high school baseball player. Athletes between the ages of 14 and 18 need more aerobic/endurance work than college and pro athletes, who are more physically mature.

Conditioning Drills

The key to creating any conditioning drill is adhering to the proper work to rest/active rest ratios. A 1:3–5 work to rest ratio is best for the game of baseball.

In practical terms:

1:3 work to rest ratio
10 seconds work : 30 seconds of rest
6 seconds work : 18 seconds of rest

1:4 work to rest ratio
8 seconds work : 32 seconds of rest
4 seconds work : 16 seconds of rest

1:5 work to rest ratio
8 seconds work : 40 seconds of rest
4 seconds work : 20 seconds of rest

Of course, these ratios are best used as guidelines. Rarely do head coaches run a practice according to a stopwatch, so the key is to use a few pre-planned drills that you know will take advantage of proper work to rest ratios.

Real World Advice: Put kids into groups of 3, 4, 5 to create natural work to rest ratios.

When creating and choosing the best conditioning drills, keep it simple and specific to the game of baseball.

- 5–15 yard linear sprints to build acceleration

- 30–60 yard linear sprints to build full speed

- 5–10 yard shuttles to build change of direction and eccentric strength

- 30–60 yard circle sprints to build max speed on the bases

Combine these drills with the above work-to-rest ratio while using multiple start positions (push-up starts, lunge starts, and base stealing starts) and you have an endless number of combinations.

On-Field Conditioning Drills

Acceleration	10 yard chase sprints from a lunge position (inside leg up)	All players line up on the right field line in a lunge position with one player placed 1–2 yards ahead of the others. The sprint starts on the coach's "GO." The other players must attempt to catch the player in front. Walk back to the line for active rest, 6–10 reps.
Acceleration	10 yard chase sprints from a lunge position (outside leg up)	All players line up on the right field line in a lunge position with one player placed 1–2 yards ahead of the others. The sprint starts on the coach's "GO." The other players must attempt to catch the player in front. Walk back to the line for active rest, 6–10 reps.
Repeat Sprint Ability	60 yard chase sprint from a push-up (down) start	All players line up on the right field line in a push-up position with one player designated as "offense." The player on "offense" may sprint at will; the remaining players must react to his first movement and sprint to catch him, 4–8 reps.
Repeat Sprint Ability	30 yard chase sprint from a push-up start	All players line up on the right field line in a down push-up position with one player designated on "offense" in an up push-up position. The player on "offense" may sprint at will; the remaining players must react to his first movement and sprint to catch him, 4–8 reps.
Short Shuttle	Competition Pro Agility (5-10-5) Drill	Two players line up facing each other at the middle cone. One is designated "offense" and can sprint at will; the remaining players must react to his first movement and sprint to catch him, 6–10 reps.
Circle Repeat Sprint Ability	60 yard circle chase sprint in a forward lunge position	Set up a circle of cones about 60 yards long in the outfield with two players lined up at the first cone in a lunge position with one player placed 3–5 yards ahead of the other. The sprint starts on the coach's "GO." Walk back to the line for active rest, 3–6 reps in each direction.

Weight Room Conditioning Drills

Aerobic Capacity	Continuous Bike Work	20–40 minutes on a stationary bike at about 60–70% of your maximum heart rate can build your aerobic base. This is best for pitchers the day after a start in-season.
Repeat Sprint Ability	10-yard Sled Push	Push a sled with 90–180 lbs. (based on your strength and conditioning levels) for 10 yards. Working in groups of 3–4 creates a natural work to rest ratio. Work up to 10 sprints.
High Intensity (Anaerobic) Conditioning	Multi Station Circuit Training #1	Circuit training options are limited only to your facility and creativity. Here is one of my favorites: 6–8 rounds of 15 seconds work and 45 seconds rest 1A. Sideboard lateral slides 1B. Step up jumps on a 12-inch box 1C. Fan bike sprints 1D. Incline treadmill sprints 1E. Jump rope
High Intensity (Anaerobic) Conditioning	Multi Station Circuit Training #2	6–8 rounds of 15 seconds work and 45 seconds rest 1A. Fan bike sprints 1B. Lunge jumps 1C. Plyo (clap) push ups 1D. 250 meter erg/rower 1E. Single leg jump rope (alternate every 5 jumps)
High Intensity (Anaerobic) Conditioning	Dumbbell Complex	Complexes are essentially high intensity circuits, but using only one piece of equipment. 2–3 rounds for 8 reps each exercise with 2–3 minutes of rest between rounds 1A. Dumbbell Single Arm Snatch 1B. Dumbbell Shoulder Press 1C. Dumbbell Sumo Deadlift 1D. Dumbbell Row 1E. Dumbbell Squat Jump

Pay attention to your work to rest ratios and try to incorporate the majority of your conditioning into your practice time. A well-run practice can be all the conditioning a position player needs.

A FINAL WORD ON SPEED DEVELOPMENT VS. CONDITIONING

Speed is *not* conditioning. Speed can only be truly developed if you allow athletes a full recovery between reps. Sprinting is an explosive movement, and must be trained as such…which is why I program the majority of sprint workouts by putting the players in a position of competition. Everyone runs faster when they are chasing, or being chased; if you allow your athletes full recovery between reps and then ask them for their best effort, they *will* get faster. Conditioning on the other hand, is putting the body into a position of fatigue for the purposes of improved recovery and stamina. Essentially, speed and conditioning drills can be very similar, but their drill distances, intensities, and rest intervals set them apart.

PITCHER-SPECIFIC CONDITIONING

Pitchers follow a very similar work-to-rest ratio as the position players, with the only difference being a guaranteed larger volume of work. A position player may only have to make a few plays or run the bases (we hope) a few times each game. That is why the focus for all position players is speed. To give a gross generalization, pitchers average 15 pitches per game and no two innings are the same. Therefore, typically pitchers—and only pitchers—need to be able to handle a higher volume on a weekly basis.

Run Timed Sprints!

In the last few years, I have added year-round (6–10 reps per week) 10-yard sprints (Acceleration) and 10-yard flying sprints (Speed) with a Brower Timing Laser System. We test for three reasons:

1. Running timed sprints gives the kids a **chance to compete.**
2. The sprints **measure the progress** of their training.
3. The sprints also **measure recovery.**

"Recovery equals stress" comes in all forms. Once I have a baseline, if Athlete A runs a full tenth of a second or 0.2 seconds SLOWER, he/she is probably under-recovered. This metric allows me to adjust the workout and program in a workout designed for recovery. If Athlete A runs a tenth of a second or 0.05 seconds FASTER, that's awesome! A new PR! They can attack the workout that day.

Please refer to Les Spellman, Tony Holler, and Mike Boyle on how to make timed sprint affordable and effective.

RECOVERY STRATEGIES

We all want to train hard, but we often forget the need for equal effort in our recovery—which is why injuries are on the rise. A simple Google search for "youth baseball pitching injuries" yields about 55,600,000 results, which gives you an idea of how this phenomenon affects younger athletes in particular.

Overuse injuries can be defined as "an imbalance caused by overly intensive training and inadequate recovery." Experts are now seeing an increase in some of the more severe overuse injuries in younger patients, including a sharp increase in the number of young athletes requiring reconstructive elbow surgery (commonly known as Tommy John surgery).

An athlete's ability to recover is crucial. It allows them to train more frequently, harder, longer, and continue their fitness pursuits.

Bottom line? **Faster recovery = better performance.**

PREVENTING OVERUSE INJURIES IN BASEBALL

According to renowned orthopedic sports surgeon Dr. James Andrews, overuse injuries—especially those related to the UCL and shoulder—*are* preventable. Some tips to keep you in the game throughout your life include:

- Warm up properly by stretching, running, and easy, gradual throwing

- Rotate playing to other positions besides pitcher

- Concentrate on age-appropriate pitching

- Develop skills that are age appropriate and adhere to pitch count guidelines, such as those established by Little League Baseball

- Avoid pitching on multiple teams with overlapping seasons

- Don't pitch through elbow or shoulder pain; if pain persists, see a doctor

- Don't pitch on consecutive days and don't play year-round

- Never use a radar gun

- Communicate regularly about how your arm is feeling and if there is any pain

- Emphasize control, accuracy, and good mechanics; master the fastball first and the change-up second, before considering breaking pitches

- Speak with a sports medicine professional or athletic trainer if you have any concerns about injuries or prevention strategies

Remember, arm care takes on many different forms. Adhering to the above list is certainly a factor; it also includes following the Pitch Smart program created by USA Baseball and MLB. Pitch Smart is a series of practical, age-appropriate guidelines to help parents, players and coaches avoid overuse injuries and foster long, healthy careers for youth pitchers. The "arm care" exercises found in this are very humbling—done correctly, even a 3 or 5 lbs. dumbbell will have never felt so heavy!

SLEEP

Sleep may be the most important factor in boosting recovery ability. Athletes should be in bed by 10 pm (which means shutting down all screens and devices well before that) and get 8–10 hours of sleep per night. Good sleep is more potent than any dietary supplement you can pick up at GNC! A lack of sleep can also impede your ability to lose weight.

Some good sleep tips include:

- Black out your room to boost melatonin levels

- Use a meditation app

- Maintain a regular bedtime and wake-up time

- Develop a regular bedtime routine just as you would a consistent pre-game routine

- Use ear plugs

- Make a to-do list for tomorrow's tasks and activities before getting into bed in order to minimize stress

Sleep has become such a point of emphasis at the professional level that organizations now employ a sleep doctor as a consultant for players who need help with sleeping at all levels, whether it be things like just staying asleep, adjusting to time zone changes, or sleeping on buses.

LIFTING

Light muscle activation increases blood flow and speeds up recovery. That is why the best prescription for soreness is light activity.

The best light activities are:

- **Sled workouts.** Load your pulling sled with light weight, just enough to get the blood flowing. Sleds are particularly effective due to the dynamic stretching and lack of eccentric loading involved.

- **Bodyweight workouts.** Jumping rope, squats, walking lunges, push-ups, TRX row, and band pull-aparts are all great body weight workouts for light activation. Try for 2 sets of 10–15 reps each exercise.

- **Fan bike workouts.** Full body cardio for 20–30 minutes at 60 percent of your max heart rate will really get blood flowing.

HYDRATION

A dehydrated athlete cramps and suffers from poor performance. Try to drink ¾–1 ounce of water per pound of body weight each day.

NUTRITION

As mentioned, eating more protein helps fuel muscle recovery. Directly after your workout, try to eat 20–40 grams of protein to jump start the recovery process. Also, eat a good breakfast to get your metabolism going.

SELF MYOFASCIAL RELEASE (SMR)

The foam roller is the most popular choice for this type of post-workout release. Daily or twice-daily massages of the muscles will greatly help recovery by enhancing blood flow and breaking down scar tissue built up during tough workouts.

Other SMR tools include:

- Lacrosse ball
- Tennis ball or yoga tune up balls
- Foam roller, homemade PVC foam roller, or Rumble Roller
- The Stick
- TriggerPoint's Performance Kit

PREHAB EXERCISES

Perhaps the most overlooked and important aspect of recovery is avoiding damage by preventing overuse. Prehab exercises are movements that strength coaches have borrowed from physical therapists (PT) and athletic trainers (ATC) for healthy athletes. Essentially, prehab is rehab exercise done while healthy in order to prevent injury. The most overused areas for baseball players are the knees, hips, and shoulders. Some of my favorite prehab exercises for dealing with these problem areas include:

Knee Prehab

- Strength Band TKE (Terminal Knee Extension)

- Foam Roll IT Band

- Stability Ball Single Leg Glute Bridge

Hip Prehab

- Bulgarian Squat Stretch

- Cook Hip Lift

- Mini Band Lateral Walks

Shoulder Prehab

- Band Pull-Aparts

- Band Side External Rotations

- 3–5 pounds Dumbbell Prone "T" Raise

HYDROTHERAPY

The pool is great for full body recovery. Pool workouts take pressure off the joints and allow for improved blood flow, improved joint range of motion, and a decrease in general muscle soreness.

Another tool is contrast showers. Post workout and post-game, cycle between hot and cold water in the shower. The contrast relaxes and excites the muscles, improves post-workout blood circulation, and shortens the restoration time.

ICING AND CRYOTHERAPY

Decreasing muscle recovery time can be done effectively with cryotherapy. The cold helps reduce inflammation and speed up the healing process. Take advantage of the ice roller, which combines the benefits of ice and foam rolling.

TESTING AND STRENGTH RATIOS

E valuation is key in any program and every exercise is an evaluation. Evaluating each athlete will help you determine the strengths and weakness of each player and help track the success of a high school strength and conditioning program over time. It also can be a huge confidence booster for younger athletes to see their scores improve as the months and years go on.

Many of the tests found in the section are also found in the IRON FALCON program on page 317. Conversely, any exercise found on the IRON FALCON program can become an area of testing.

Areas of Testing

- Movement quality

- Strength

- Power

- Speed and agility

- Organization

TESTING FOR MOVEMENT QUALITY
Deceleration (The Single Leg Hop)

The single leg hop measures any imbalance between force production (acceleration) and force absorption (deceleration) and can help determine the likelihood of a knee injury in high school athletes.

To Perform the Single Leg Hop:

- Measure a hop on your right leg for distance

- Measure a hop on your left leg for distance

- Compare the distance between each hop

Coaches should look for three issues:

1. Trouble stabilizing (or "sticking the landing")

2. A greater than 10 percent difference in distance between legs

3. Knee instability (a small amount of inward turn is acceptable for some athletes)

Failure in any of these areas typically indicates either poor hip control or a lack of deceleration and/or uneven leg strength, all of which indicate an increased injury potential.

Functional Movement (The Overhead Squat)

No one movement can reveal more imbalances within an athlete's body than the overhead squat. For best results, coaches shouldn't tell their athletes that they are being evaluated, and instead program overhead squats directly into their warm-ups to indirectly test movement quality on a weekly basis.

The overhead squat can reveal a host of overactive and underactive muscle groups, any of which can increase an athlete's chance of injury. For an extensive listing of what the overhead squat can evaluate and how to address these issues, see the National Academy of Sports Medicine's online checklist for the overhead squat. This chart was also a huge influence on the corrective exercises programmed into the activation, prehab and mobility warm-up sections of the workouts in this book.

TESTING FOR STRENGTH

The days of the 1-rep max strength test are fading away (though some head coaches still swear by them). Personally, I love Jim Wendler's 5/3/1 strength program because it provides the opportunity for new personal records with each day's "+" set. Instead of constantly striving for a new one rep max, work for a new REP MAX. For example, you got stronger when you increased your reps from 3 to 6 with 85 lbs. on the Goblet Bulgarian Squat.

The best tests for strength are the exercises that make the foundation of your program. For me, it is the barbell front squat, dumbbell bench press (or push up variation), hex bar deadlift, and the pull-up or chin-up.

THE EYE TEST

There's a lot that can be determined simply by watching athletes perform their normal strength routines, watching for any issues in form or execution. Coaches will find it extremely valuable to record all max attempts made by their players on film. If a player's max weight went up only incrementally but his movement quality has visibly improved (better depth on the squat, more stabilization at the bottom of the squat, etc.) then the players and coaches both have another tool to build up player confidence.

TESTING FOR POWER

For baseball players, this one is a no-brainer. To test for power, we look directly at the broad jump, and/or vertical jump, and the Rotational Medicine Ball Throw.

Horizontal Power (Broad Jump)

The easiest and most effective test to administer for evaluating horizontal power is the broad jump. This test directly relates to an athlete's acceleration.

To perform the broad jump test:

- Set up a tape measure

- Instruct the athlete to stand toes behind the tape measure

- Measure a jump at the heels for distance

Vertical Power

There are several methods I like to use when testing athletes for vertical power. Of these, the first two—the Vertec and the Just Jump mat—are very accurate but expensive to purchase (both units can be $650 each).

The **Vertec Jump Trainer** is the jump trainer found most often in the NBA and NFL combines. It gives immediate results, is easy to use and set up, and very accurate. It can measure standing reach and vertical leap reach. The difference between those two values is the athlete's vertical jump.

The **Just Jump Mat** is the leading choice at showcases and large group events or testing. Simply stand on the mat with your feet together and jump, and the system calculates your vertical jump height by measuring the time that your feet are not in contact with the mat. It can also calculate "hang time" for one jump, average height plus ground time for four jumps, computes explosive leg power, and can compute foot quickness (shuttle runs and dashes).

However, for those without the budget for fancy equipment, the **Old School Wall Test** is more than sufficient. Athletes will not score as high on the wall test versus the Vertec or Jump Mat, simply because they are restricted in movement having to be so close to the wall; however, it is free and easy to perform.

- Dust the athlete's fingertips with chalk

- Mark the highest point they can reach on the wall.

- Jump and mark the highest point on the wall

- Measure the distance between the marks

Regardless of the method you choose, pick one and stick with it to ensure you are comparing "apples" to "apples."

Rotational Power

Throwing a medicine ball like swinging a bat (with a shovel throw) is best way to measure rotational power.

To perform the medicine ball throw test:

- Set up a tape measure

- Instruct the athlete to stand with their front foot behind the tape measure in their hitting stance

- Using an 8–12 lbs. ball, measure the distance of the player's medicine ball throw.

- Use an under hand, shovel throw grip. Allow the athlete to finish their throw past the line to allow for max effort.

TESTING FOR SPEED AND AGILITY

When testing for speed and agility in baseball players, it's best to utilize the same tests as used in most MLB tryout camps and showcase camps: the **60-yard sprint** and the **pro agility (5-10-5) drill.**

60-Yard Sprint

This test directly measures your acceleration and top-end speed.

To perform the 60-yard Sprint:

- Measure 60 yards from the right field line

- Start standing in a two point stance facing forward

- The test starts on the athletes first movement

Pro Agility (5-10-5) Drill

This test evaluates your body control, change of direction, and lateral movement.

To perform the pro agility (5-10-5) drill:

- Set up three cones five yards apart with two tennis balls on the end lines. The tennis balls are to ensure the athletes make it to the line.

- Start on the middle cone and sprint 5 yards to your left and knock away one tennis ball.

- Change directions and sprint 10 yards to your right to knock away the other tennis ball.

- Change directions and sprint left towards the middle cone.

Remember to remain consistent in the way you test. If you hand-time sprints, for example, you must hand-time all future sprints. You cannot accurately compare hand-timed sprint results with laser-timed results.

STAYING ORGANIZED

It has never been easier to stay organized and keep track of the massive amount of valuable player data needed to accurately evaluate athletes and design programs to suit their needs. With countless programs, apps and smart devices available, it's just a matter of finding the software that works best for you and putting it to work. My choice has always been TeamBuildR. Please check out their information in the Resources section on page 326.

Not only that, but there is a wealth of information available online for coaches and players alike, including instructional videos for each exercise and routine they perform. Taking full advantage of these resources and implementing them into your program gives you more control over your progress than ever before.

STRENGTH RATIOS

It's one of the most common questions coaches hear: "What's a good weight, Coach?"

This is especially common from younger athletes still learning their way, and it's a fair question: when working with very competitive players in a very competitive environment, it's natural for athletes to want to know what their targets are. However, the problem is that each athlete is different, with different strengths and weaknesses and body frame. For example, tall athletes tend to squat and bench press less weight than their shorter teammates simply because the barbell has a longer distance to travel (longer arms and legs). Whether a player is getting stronger or not is dependent on their overall results, which take the complete athlete into account as part of the big picture.

So, how do you satisfy both these requirements?

The answer that I have found to work best is **strength ratios,** presented in two different formats:

1. Exercise Strength ratios, comparing exercise to exercise to ensure muscular balance (i.e. what are players lifting for a back squat as compared to a front squat?)

2. Body Weight Strength ratios, comparing an athlete's strength to his or her body weight (also known as relative strength)

Using the strength ratios on the following pages, players can stay balanced and finally have a satisfying answer to that eternal question of "What is a good weight?"

Each ratio is based on a foundation exercise. These numbers also provide athletes with a sense of checks and balances. This goes beyond knowing that your lower body must be stronger than your upper body. You'll benefit from taking responsibility and working on your weaknesses.

These ratios are based as much on experience as research. These numbers are for high school players, not college players or professional powerlifters. Every exercise is calculated based on a 5-rep max; male ratios are based on a body weight of 175 lbs. and female ratios are based on 125 lbs.

Baseball Relative Strength Ratios
- Barbell Back Squat at 1.5 times body weight
- Trap Bar Deadlift at 2 times body weight
- Barbell Bench Press at 1.25 times body weight
- Barbell Front Squat at 60–70% max Back Squat weight

Softball Relative Strength Ratios
- Barbell Back Squat at 1.25 times body weight
- Trap Bar Deadlift at 1.75 times body weight
- Barbell Bench Press at 75% of body weight
- Barbell Front Squat at 60–70% max Back Squat weight

As always, these are guidelines and should be adjusted to your player's abilities.

All numbers listed in the following charts are examples and should be used to illustrate the ratios.

Squat Ratios

Boys Baseball			Girls Softball		
Barbell Back Squat	5 rep max	235	Barbell Back Squat	5 rep max	140
Barbell Front Squat	60%	145	Barbell Front Squat	60%	85
	70%	165		70%	100
Barbell Deadlift	110%	260	Barbell Deadlift	110%	155
	120%	285		120%	170
Barbell RDL	70%	185	Barbell RDL	70%	110
Barbell Glute Bridge	100%	235	Barbell Glute Bridge	100%	140

Push players to be able to front squat at a ratio of 60–70% of their back squat. This shows a balance of core stability, posterior chain strength, and thoracic spine mobility. Players may deadlift slightly more weight than their squat because of their limb length and ankle mobility restrictions.

Deadlift Ratios

Boys Baseball			Girls Softball		
Trap Bar Deadlift	5 rep max	305	Trap Bar Deadlift	5 rep max	195
Barbell Deadlift	85%	260	Barbell Deadlift	85%	170
	90%	275		90%	180
Barbell RDL	70%	185	Barbell RDL	70%	120
Trap Bar Jump Squat	30%	95	Trap Bar Jump Squat	30%	60
Trap Bar Jump Shrug	60%	185	Trap Bar Jump Shrug	60%	120
Barbell Hang Clean	60%	160	Barbell Hang Clean	60%	105

As this is based on a 5-rep max trap bar deadlift, players may end up lifting 10–15 percent less on the conventional deadlift because it is a much more difficult lift. To maintain balance, players will want to perform RDLs at about 70 percent of their deadlift. This shows a good balance of core stability and hamstring flexibility.

In regard to power development, we want players to hang clean for 60 percent of their deadlift. These numbers may seem conservative, but when coaching barbell speed and higher (1/4 squat) catch positions we want to maximize athleticism and power production and minimize lower back injuries.

Bench Press Ratios

Boys Baseball			Girls Softball		
Dumbbell Bench Press	5 rep max	65	Dumbbell Bench Press	5 rep max	30
Dumbbell Incline Bench Press	70%	45	Dumbbell Incline Bench Press	70%	17.5
	80%	55		80%	20
Dumbbell Shoulder Press	60%	35	Dumbbell Shoulder Press	60%	15
Dumbbell Push Press	70%	45	Dumbbell Push Press	70%	20

The weights listed are for a single dumbbell. Players must grab a pair of dumbbells for the exercise. Players should push to within 70–80 percent of their max dumbbell bench press for the incline bench press. I coach our players to use a neutral grip on all dumbbell pressing for safe and healthy shoulders. I set the incline to 15–30 degrees for incline bench press.

Most importantly, players need to be able to shoulder press at about 60 percent of their bench press. This shows a good balance of horizontal and vertical pressing.

Finally, you could easily exchange the dumbbell bench press for the any variation of push up. I ask for 2–3 sets of 25 push-ups from the boys and 2–3 sets of 10-15 push-ups from the girls.

FINAL WORD ON STRENGTH RATIOS

These ratios are the backboard for the creation of the IRON FALCON program (page 317). The IRON FALCON program was created to generate healthy competition in the weight room, using quantifiable athletic movements that will give athletes the physical tools to become baseball players.

SQUAT AND DEADLIFT CONSIDERATIONS FOR TALLER ATHLETES

As mentioned earlier, there are a few unique aspects to consider when applying averaged strength ratios to taller players with longer limbs. Make sure your players are bearing these in mind, to avoid any potential confusion or discouragement.

- Taller players with longer arms and legs will have trouble getting down to parallel due to simply having a greater distance to travel (compared to shorter players).
- Longer levers (arms and legs) are harder to control and require more joint stability.
- Restrictions in thoracic spine (T-spine) mobility must be addressed to ensure proper posture and to avoid lower back pain.
- Ankle sprains lead to scar tissue. Scar tissue leads to a decreased range of motion and lack of mobility. Keep in mind any athlete with an injury history of ankle sprains. If a joint (ankle in this case) cannot achieve a certain range of motion during a deep squat, the surrounding joints will be overloaded. If you have consistent lower back pain after squat day, double check your ankle mobility.
- Adhere to the squat progressions on page 74 and deadlift progressions on page 70 to allow for body weight competency first. You never want to load dysfunction.
- Place a higher box under an athlete to minimize squat depth while you are working on ankle mobility and core stability. Similarly, raise the barbell off the ground (4–6 inches) with blocks during deadlift to allow a more upright posture while you work on core stability and hip hinge practice.
- Maintain a vertical shin to mitigate additional shearing forces on the knee.
- Exercises like the box squat, dumbbell goblet squat, deadlift, sumo deadlift, and lunges can allow for a more vertical shin and maybe help support your knees' long term health.
- One caveat to the vertical shin: You cannot completely throw out the traditional deep squat pattern because you will start to lose dynamic ankle mobility. Make sure to continue to use at least the body weight squat, frog squat, toe touch squat, dumbbell goblet squat in your warmup, mobility, or prehab routines.

INTENSITY TECHNIQUES

When looking to increase the intensity of your workouts, it helps to consider the top three training factors for boosting muscle growth:

1. **Mechanical tension**
2. **Muscle damage**
3. **Metabolic stress**

MECHANICAL TENSION (MAX LIFTING)

By altering your body's leverage or adding an external load to increase the force on a specific muscle through a full range of motion, you increase the amount of mechanical tension on the muscle and improve the workout. For example, by shifting your body from a 45-degree body angle to parallel to the ground during a Suspension Trainer Push-Up or Row or adding additional plates to your deadlift, you increase the tension of the workout.

MUSCLE DAMAGE (SLOW NEGATIVES)

By keeping constant tension on a muscle during an extended number of reps (also called "time under tension") you increase the degree of microtears in the muscle, thus improving the amount of muscle gained during recovery. For example, you can increase muscle damage by never locking out your elbows at the top or the bottom of a bench or by simply adding reps and sets (volume). The eccentric and isometric-based training discussed in the Building Deceleration in the Weight Room section is another great example.

METABOLIC STRESS: CHASING "THE PUMP"

In applying the concept of metabolic stress to a workout, the important elements are slow negatives and exercise variety. Slow negatives means increasing the amount of time spent in the movement, such as taking 5 seconds to lower yourself during a push-up (as opposed to the standard 1–2 seconds). Exercise variety, as the name implies, would be switching from the standard Bench Press to the Incline Bench Press, or any number of exercise variations as shown in the Progression/Advancement chart on page 65.

ADDITIONAL INTENSITY TECHNIQUES

These add variety and brutal effectiveness to any of the foundational movements. While some of these techniques are programmed into the workouts in this book, they can all be used when you feel your team's regimen is getting stale.

Drop Sets. Take a set to failure with a weight, then immediately do another set to failure with a lighter weight. As a basic rule-of-thumb, reduce the weight by around 10 percent with each drop.

Mechanical Drop Sets. Instead of simply dropping the weight to continue the set, you "drop" to an exercise with more mechanical advantage. (For example: moving from a shoulder press to a chest press to continue the set or a pull-up to ring row.)

Rack and Run. Choose a weight and take it to failure at 6-8 reps. Rack those weights and grab a set 5 pounds lighter (if using fixed dumbbells) or pull the pin and go 10 pounds lighter if using power blocks. Take that new weight to failure and repeat the process until you're holding 10 pounds in your hands. This is a classic finisher for isolation exercises like shoulder raise and biceps curl.

Elevator Set. A subset of the mechanical drop set, but now going down the elevator. Starting with a shoulder press, progress to a flat bench press in 3–5 sets, no rest, with the same weight.

Ladders. Progressively add weight with each set, taking short rest periods until you reach your max weight for 8 reps. Then, go back down in weight each set until you reach the original weight.

Cluster Sets. Break down one set into multiple mini-sets. To do this, lift your 6-rep max for 3 reps for multiple sets (2–4) with only 10–20 seconds of rest between sets. The goal is to lift the same weight for all three sets and get more total reps at the specific weight than a traditional straight set. While we suggest you have a spotter for every exercise, you really must have a spotter for cluster sets.

Rest/Pause Sets. This is a variation of cluster sets, now using a 10-rep max weight for a set of 8 reps with 20–25 seconds of rest for 3 sets. This technique breaks down one traditional strength set into multiple mini-sets, and is itself a variation of cluster sets. With only a few, well timed, short breaks within a set, you are able to get more reps at a specific weight. The difference between a cluster set and a rest/pause set is that, in a rest/pause set, you lift a weight closer to your max to failure each set, with your reps decreasing each successive set (because of the shorter rest periods) and going until muscle failure each set.

Pre-Exhaust Sets. Do a set of isolation exercises for a muscle group; then, with no rest, do a compound movement of the same muscle group. This is an old school body building technique.

Density Training. The goal is to perform as many reps of your chosen movement or movements as possible in a given period of time. Start easy with about 5 minutes and work your way up to a 10-15 minute round. These are great to finish a workout when you're pressed for time.

Circuits. A series of exercises done in succession without rest, done for time or reps. Permutations are endless. This style of training has been around for years and has recently taken on the name metabolic resistance training (MRT). These are super effective in the off-season for athletes looking to drop body fat.

Complexes. These are essentially circuits with one piece of equipment (barbell, dumbbell, sandbag, medicine ball, or a 45 lbs. weight plate). The options are endless. They are also brutally effective for off-season conditioning, to keep athletes mentally fresh when they need a change of pace in the weight room, and to build grip strength.

Post Activation Potentiation (PAP) Sets. This method is a go-to for many high-level athletes. Essentially, you pair a heavy compound exercise (dumbbell chest press, for example) with a lighter, dynamic exercise (such as plyometric push-ups). By combining a strength exercise at 75–85 percent of max, immediately followed by a similar power exercise, you build explosive power.

Super Sets. This pairs two exercises with no rest. Variations on the super set are endless, but my favorites are:

- Sets within the same muscle (back to back chest exercises)
  - Ex. Push-Ups/Dips

- Sets with opposing muscles (hamstring and quad exercises)
  - Ex. Leg Curl/Squat

- Sets with opposing upper body/lower body exercises
  - Ex. Row/Reverse Lunge

PSD Sets. Utilizes the old school bodybuilding techniques of a pre-exhaust set, a strength set, and a mechanical drop set.

747 Sets. These sets help increase work capacity by building power and endurance. These are very tough and will challenge even the strongest high school athletes. Beginning with 7 reps using a moderate weight, and without resting, increase the load and complete 4 reps. Finish the set by doing another 7 reps using a lighter weight.

Dynamic Effort (DE) Sets. Dynamic effort sets build strength and speed by working at a moderate intensity (55–70 percent) with max bar speed for only 2–3 reps for 8–10 sets.

Max Effort (RE) Sets. This is your traditional strength training set-up, working at high intensity (80–100 percent of max) for 1–5 reps and 3–8 sets.

Repetition Effort (RE) Sets. These sets are inspired by powerlifting legend Louie Simmons and his conjugate method. Repetition effort builds massive size by working at a moderate intensity (65–75 percent) for only higher volumes of 8–12 reps for 3–5 sets.

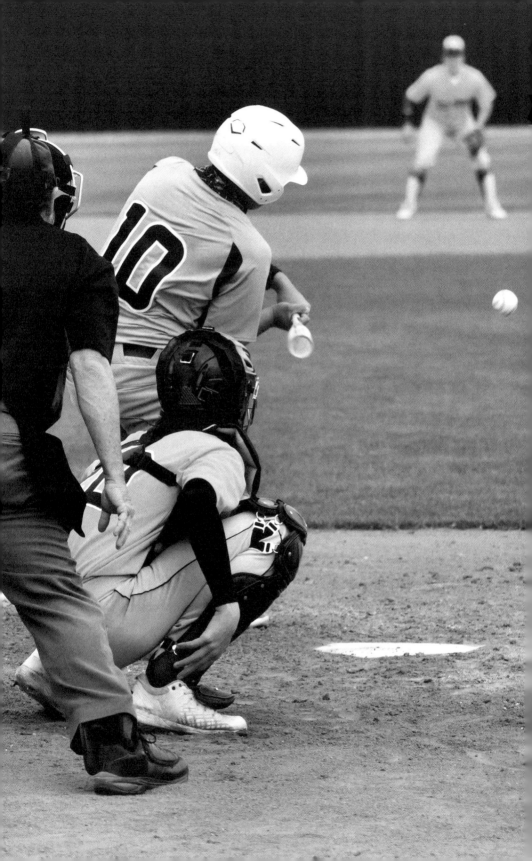

THE WORKOUTS

S trength, power and speed are the factors that determine who is a starter, and who is a nonstarter—who is JV, and who is varsity.

This book covers the following phases of player development:

1. Freshman and JV levels
2. Varsity baseball

This book also covers a full year—four seasons of training—for the varsity player:

1. In Season (Spring)
2. Post-Season (Summer)
3. Off Season (Fall)
4. Pre-Season (Winter)

FRESHMAN TO JV LEVEL

Just as a freshman student would initially enroll in a "level 100" subject course class in preparation for further study of the same subject in an "advanced" level setting, it is also necessary to physically prepare the high school athlete for the eventual implementation of advanced exercises and higher intensities prior to their actual application. The Freshman to JV level workouts are all about building up a player's foundation, making sure that they're properly prepared in terms of mobility, endurance, and strength to perform at the level expected of a varsity athlete.

THE GOAL: "FRESHMAN AND JV PLAYERS MUST EARN THE BARBELL"

In the programs I design, I place prerequisites that need to be completed before any player is granted the privilege of using the barbell. This is a "slow roast" approach, which is essential in any high school player's development. Granted, some of the younger players may "earn the barbell" in their first few weeks of training; nevertheless, this process builds a culture of working hard to earn your place, both on the team and in the weight room.

Coaching Point

You will have to adjust for your bigger players who are new to the weight room. A taller and/or heavier player who cannot do one push-up and is embarrassed to try would absolutely benefit from learning the Dumbbell Bench Press before push-ups. Alternately, being a heavier player makes it difficult to stay true to the percentages outlined below.

For example, a 205 lbs. boy new to the weight room would be asked for a 100 lbs. Dumbbell Goblet Squat and Kettlebell Sumo Deadlift before "earning the barbell," which is simply not feasible. Same for a 160 lbs. girl: technically, she would be asked for an 80 lbs. Dumbbell Goblet Squat and Kettlebell Sumo Deadlift—not realistic at all.

When I have a taller and/or heavier athlete new to the weight room, I assign them fixed goals for the Dumbbell Goblet Squat and Kettlebell Sumo Deadlift first. At minimum, all athletes must Dumbbell Goblet Squat and Kettlebell Sumo Deadlift 45 or 50 lbs. (which is what the barbell and hex bar weigh). This avoids the embarrassment of never accomplishing an unrealistic goal and allows them to naturally progress with their teammates, as well as avoids potential safety issues. This directly relates back to the "art of coaching" on page 5.

In order to perform a Barbell Front Box Squat, a player must be able to perform a Dumbbell Goblet Squat for 20 reps at half their body weight.

VARSITY BASEBALL

Our training program, and all the workouts in this book, are broken down to match the four seasons of the school year. Each phase (season) of training includes seasonal specific workouts, outlined below. I also provide a general goal and theme for each phase to keep the athlete focused and on task. While every school calendar is different, this is a workout schedule that most high school players can identify with. Please adjust as needed according to your school calendar, baseball game schedule, and academic load.

In-Season: Spring (March to June)
Athlete Focus: Stay Strong and Injury Free

During the in-season, we expect all varsity level athletes to train twice a week following a total body program. These workouts are a smaller version (fewer reps, sets, and training sessions) than their pre-season winter workouts, with a greater focus on shoulder prehab to allow for complete recovery and forearm strength so that they are in top shape for game day. The lifting during the season is just as crucial to performance as the off-season workouts because the games at the end of the season are just as, if not more, important than those at the start of the year. So if all of your hard work goes to waste because you didn't train to stay strong for the whole season, then why train in the off-season?

Post-Season: Summer (June to July)
Athlete Focus: Rebuild Strength

During this 4-week general physical preparation (GPP) phase, we program for some variation of the "Big 5." We focus on re-building stability and building a solid range of motion after a grueling season, including teaching and practicing the front squat position. We don't do any dynamic work (jumping or medicine ball work) or sprint work, and minimize the load on the barbell to allow for further recovery in the early spring. These are a very important 4 weeks that set the table for injury-free strength and power training in the following summer months.

Off-Season I: Summer (July and August)
Athlete Focus: Build Strength

Coming off the GPP phase and heading into the summer months, we build on the "Big 5" with a focus on eccentric and isometric work while striving to build size and strength with four lift days per week (two upper body and two lower body). This is your best opportunity to build strength in preparation for next season.

Off-Season II: Fall (September to Thanksgiving Break)
Athlete Focus: Build Strength, Power, and Speed

Transitioning from the off-season program, the next phase puts greater emphasis on power and strength development. You move back to three workout sessions per week to allow for fall baseball and schoolwork. Some players may need to take a complete break from training (weight room and baseball) for the second half of this phase due to coming off of a six month competitive season. (see below).

THE SHOWCASE AND TRAVEL BALL EFFECT

After the high school season, some players move right into travel ball for the summer and fall season, which must be taken into account when programming an athlete's workouts. During the summer months while playing travel baseball, athletes may be able to dedicate more time to training and recovery—enough to allow for four workouts per week. Depending on the frequency of travel and distance to tournaments, three full-body training sessions per week may be best.

Finally, if athletes played competitive baseball from March/April to October/November (depending on where you live), they must take a few weeks to physically and mentally recharge (this is typically in August for most competitive baseball players). Therefore, you could do the post-season rebuild strength program workouts again to prepare for the winter pre-season program.

I provide three days a week, four days a week, and five days a week program options that focus on strength, power, and speed, that you can use to best fit your schedule. Remember, consistent hard work is more important than the perfect program.

Pre-Season: Winter (Mid-November to February)

Athlete Focus: Build Explosiveness and Speed

Workouts in the weight room begin to rotate, focusing on strength, size, and power, in what is known as daily undulating periodization (DUP). Workout days dedicated to speed and power development focus on acceleration, change of direction, reaction agility, and team competition drills.

FRESHMAN/JV LEVEL

U nlike varsity athletes, freshman and JV player workouts are *not* seasonal. Freshman/JV level workouts focus on the building blocks of strength: mobility, core stability, and exercises to build up to the varsity "Big 5" and the 10 foundational movements. For that reason, we focus training the entire body every time in the weight room. This program is a 4-week, 12-workout phase that is not specific to any season. It is very similar to the varsity player's post-season phases, in that both are general physical preparation (GPP) based.

At this early stage, athletes cannot handle the same volume (reps, set, and load) of training as varsity players. The focus *cannot* be on heavy weights, it must be learning the *skill* of movement. Pushing an exercise to muscle failure at this age can be dangerous. Many of these athletes are in the weight room for the first time. In order to learn a new skill, an athlete must be allowed a chance to practice (frequency), with body control (avoid muscle fatigue), and proper technique (no technical failure).

Credit goes to Zach Dechant and his book *Movement Over Maxes*. His chapter on the principles of the foundation program was a "lightbulb" moment for me in allowing younger athletes the chance learn a new skill in the weight room with more (sometime daily) training frequency. We let 12-year-olds play 3-5 games in a weekend; therefore, do not overreact to a player getting in the gym every day for a supervised workout.

Program Breakdown

Day 1	Day 2	Day 3
Target Area: Mobility	**Target Area:** Mobility	**Target Area:** Mobility
Target Area: Core Stability	**Target Area:** Core Stability	**Target Area:** Core Stability
Tier 2: Throw	**Tier 2:** Rotation	**Tier 2:** Jump
Tier 1: Deadlift	**Tier 1:** Pull-Up	**Tier 1:** Squat
Tier 2: Lunge	**Tier 2:** Carry	**Tier 1:** Chin-Up
Tier 1: Bench Press	**Tier 2:** Lunge	**Tier 3:** Posterior Chain
Target Area: Forearm	**Target Area:** Shoulder	**Target Area:** Forearm

PROGRAM NOTES

- Please follow these workouts in order. They have been programmed to progress based on having successfully completed the previous workout.

- The mobility and core stability exercises given are at a varsity level, to give younger athletes an accurate goal to work towards.

- The overall volume (reps multiplied by sets) given is lower than varsity workouts.

- These workouts are based on the Progression/Advancement chart given on page 65–66.

- Dedicated and motivated players can certainly do another two days in the weight room learning and practicing the skills of a new exercise, provided they keep it to body weight exercise only and limit the reps to 5 and sets to 2–3.

WEEK 1
Foundation Workout #1

Target Area: Mobility
Band Overhead Squat Pattern - 2 sets of 10 reps
Dumbbell "T" Balance - 2 sets of 8 reps per leg

Target Area: Core Stability
Plank - 2 sets of 60 seconds
Side Plank - 2 sets of 45 seconds per side

Tier 2: Throw
Medicine Ball Scoop Throw - 3 sets of 5 reps

Tier 1: Deadlift
Dumbbell Goblet Box Squat - 3 sets of 8–12 reps

Tier 2: Lunge
Body Weight Split Squat - 2 sets of 15 reps per leg

Tier 1: Bench Press
Push-Ups - 3 sets of 15 reps

Target Area: Forearm
Dumbbell Wrist Extension - 3 sets of 10 reps each

ALL SEASONAL

FRESHMAN/JV LEVEL

WEEK 1
Foundation Workout #2

Target Area: Mobility
Band Pull-Aparts - 2 sets of 15–20 reps
Wall Half Kneeling 3-Way Ankle Mobility - 2 sets of 5 per leg

Target Area: Core Stability
Alternate Leg Raise - 2 sets of 10 reps per leg
Back Extension ISO (Holds) - 2 sets of 60 seconds

Tier 2: Rotation
Standing Cable Lift - 2 sets of 8 reps per side

Tier 1: Pull-Up
Suspension Training (TRX or Rings) Row - 3 sets of 15 reps

Tier 2: Carry
Dumbbell Single Arm Farmer Walk - 3 sets of 30 yards per direction

Tier 2: Lunge
Body Weight Reverse Lunge - 2 sets of 15 reps per leg

Target Area: Shoulder
Band Pull-Aparts - 2 sets of 15 reps

WEEK 1
Foundation Workout #3

Target Area: Mobility
Dumbbell "T" Raise (Rear Delt Raise) - 2 sets of 15 reps
Foam Roll (Lat Muscles) - 2 sets of 25 rolls

Target Area: Core Stability
Side Plank Inside Leg Raise - 2 sets of 8 reps
Dumbbell Renegade Row - 2 sets of 8 reps

Tier 2: Jump
Drop Squat - 3 sets of 8 reps

Tier 1: Squat
Dumbbell Goblet Squat - 3 sets of 8 reps

Tier 1: Chin-Up
Chin-Up Negatives (Eccentric) - 2 sets of 4 reps (1 rep = 3–5 second negative)

Tier 3: Posterior Chain
Glute Ham Bench or 45-degree Bench Back Extension - 2 sets of 15 reps

Target Area: Forearm
Barbell Wrist Curl - 2 sets of 10 reps

ALL SEASONAL

FRESHMAN/JV LEVEL

WEEK 2
Foundation Workout #4

WORKOUT PROGRESSION

- Progress to Kettlebell or Dumbbell Sumo Deadlift
- Additional reps on Split Squat
- Different push-up variation

Target Area: Mobility
Band Overhead Squat Pattern - 2 sets of 10 reps
Dumbbell "T" Balance - 2 sets of 8 reps per leg

Target Area: Core Stability
Plank - 2 sets of 60 seconds
Side Plank - 2 sets of 45 seconds per side

Tier 2: Throw
Medicine Ball Scoop Throw - 3 sets of 5 reps

Tier 1: Deadlift
Kettlebell or Dumbbell Sumo Deadlift - 3 sets of 12 reps
Kettlebell or Dumbbell Sumo Deadlift - 3 sets of 12 reps

Tier 2: Lunge
Body Weight Split Squat - 2 sets of 20 reps per leg

Tier 1: Bench Press
Push Up (feet elevated on bench) - 3 sets of 15 reps

Target Area: Forearm
Dumbbell Wrist Extension - 3 sets of 10 reps each

WEEK 2
Foundation Workout #5

WORKOUT PROGRESSION

- Progress to a more difficult body angle on the suspension row
- Heavier weight on the Farmer Walk
- More reps on Reverse Lunge

ALL SEASONAL

FRESHMAN/JV LEVEL

Target Area: Mobility
Band Pull-Aparts - 2 sets of 15–20 reps
Wall Half Kneeling 3-Way Ankle Mobility - 2 sets of 5 reps per leg

Target Area: Core Stability
Alternate Leg Raise - 2 sets of 10 reps per leg
Back Extension ISO (Holds) - 2 sets of 60 seconds

Tier 2: Rotation
Standing Cable Lift - 2 sets of 8 reps per side

Tier 1: Pull-Up
Suspension Training (TRX or Rings) Row - 3 sets of 15 reps

Tier 2: Carry
Dumbbell Single Arm Farmer Walk - 3 sets of 30 yards in each direction

Tier 2: Lunge
Body Weight Reverse Lunge - 2 sets of 20 reps per leg

Target Area: Shoulder
Band Pull-Aparts - 2 sets of 15 reps

WEEK 2
Foundation Workout #6

WORKOUT PROGRESSION

- Progress to Drop Split Squat
- Additional reps on the Goblet Squat and Back Extension

Target Area: Mobility
Dumbbell "T" Raise (Rear Delt Raise) - 2 sets of 15 reps
Foam Roll Latissimus Dorsi (Lat) Muscles - 2 sets of 25 rolls

Target Area: Core Stability
Side Plank Inside Leg Raise - 2 sets of 8 reps
Dumbbell Renegade Row - 2 sets of 8 reps

Tier 2: Jump
Drop Split Squat - 3 sets of 8 reps per leg

Tier 1: Squat
Dumbbell Goblet Squat - 3 sets of 12 reps

Tier 1: Chin-Up
Chin-Up Negatives (Eccentric) - 2 sets of 4 reps (1 rep = 3–5 second negative)

Tier 3: Posterior Chain
Glute Ham Bench OR 45-degree bench Back Extension - 2 sets of 20 reps

Target Area: Forearm
Barbell Wrist Curl - 2 sets of 10 reps

WEEK 3
Foundation Workout #7

WORKOUT PROGRESSION

- New Tier 2: Throw exercise
- Use heavier weight on Sumo Deadlift
- Additional reps on the Push-Up

ALL SEASONAL

FRESHMAN/JV LEVEL

Target Area: Mobility
Prisoner Frog Squat - 3 sets of 12 reps
PVC Bench Thoracic Extension - 3 sets of 30–45 seconds

Target Area: Core Stability
Physioball Dead Bug - 3 sets of 8 super slow reps
Side Plank - 3 sets of 45 seconds per side

Tier 2: Throw
Medicine Ball Reverse Scoop Throw - 3 sets of 5 reps

Tier 1: Deadlift
Kettlebell or Dumbbell Sumo Deadlift - 3 sets of 12 reps

Tier 2: Lunge
Body Weight Split Squat - 3 sets of 20 reps per leg

Tier 1: Bench Press
Push-Ups - 3 sets of 20 reps

Target Area: Forearm
Dumbbell Wrist Extension - 3 sets of 10 reps each

WEEK 3
Foundation Workout #8

WORKOUT PROGRESSION

- Progress to Pull-Up Negatives
- Heavier weight on the Farmer Walk
- Add weight to the Reverse Lunge
- Increase volume on Shoulder exercise

Target Area: Mobility
ISO Front Squat - 3 sets of 20 seconds
Band Overhead Squat Pattern - 3 sets of 12 reps

Target Area: Core Stability
Push-Up Plank with Alternate Arm Raise - 3 sets of 12 reps per arm
Alternate Leg Raise Circles - 3 sets of 6 reps per leg, per direction

Tier 2: Rotation
Standing Cable Lift - 2 sets of 8 reps per side

Tier 1: Pull-Up
Pull-Up Negatives (Eccentric) - 2 sets of 4 reps (1 rep = 3–5 seconds negative)

Tier 2: Carry
Dumbbell Single Arm Farmer Walk - 3 sets of 30 yards in each direction

Tier 2: Lunge
Dumbbell Goblet Reverse Lunge - 2 sets of 12 reps per leg

Target Area: Shoulder
Band Pull-Aparts - 3 sets of 15 reps

WEEK 3
Foundation Workout #9

WORKOUT PROGRESSION

- Progress to Depth Drop off Short Box
- Additional reps of Chin-Up Negatives
- Attempt Glute Ham Raise this week

ALL SEASONAL

Target Area: Mobility
Single Leg Glute Bridge - 3 sets of 10 reps per leg
Kneeling Thoracic Rotations - 3 sets of 10 reps per side

Target Area: Core Stability
Physioball Front Plank Circles - 3 sets of 30–45 seconds
Alternate Leg Raise - 3 sets of 10 reps per leg

FRESHMAN/JV LEVEL

Tier 2: Jump
Depth Drop off Short Box - 3 sets of 8 reps

Tier 1: Squat
Dumbbell Goblet Squat - 3 sets of 12 reps

Tier 1: Chin-Up
Chin-Up Negatives (Eccentric) - 2 sets of 6 reps (1 rep = 3–5 second Negative)

Tier 3: Posterior Chain
Try Glute Ham Raise - 2 sets of 8 reps
If not, try Slider Leg Curl or 45-degree Bench Back Extension - 2 sets of 20 reps

Target Area: Forearm
Barbell Wrist Curl - 2 sets of 10 reps

WEEK 4
Foundation Workout #10

WORKOUT PROGRESSION

- New Tier 2: Throw exercise
- Attempt a Kettlebell or Dumbbell Sumo Deadlift (up to 100 pounds); attempt High Handle Trap Bar Deadlift if confident
- Progress to Bulgarian Squat and Suspension Trainer Push-Up

Target Area: Mobility
Foam Roll Latissimus Dorsi (Lat) Muscles - 3 sets of 20 rolls
Medicine Ball Thoracic Extension - 3 sets of 6 deep breaths

Target Area: Core Stability
Physioball Dead Bug - 3 sets of 8 reps (performed slowly)
Side Plank - 3 sets of 45 seconds per side

Tier 2: Throw
Medicine Ball Squat and Press Throw - 3 sets of 5 reps

Tier 1: Deadlift
Kettlebell or Dumbbell Sumo Deadlift - 3 sets of 12 reps

Tier 2: Lunge
Body Weight Bulgarian Squat - 2 sets of 20 reps per leg

Tier 1: Bench Press
Suspension Trainer Push-Up - 2 sets of 20 reps
Hands on the handles, feet on the floor.

Target Area: Forearm
Dumbbell Wrist Extension - 3 sets of 10 reps each

WEEK 4
Foundation Workout #11

WORKOUT PROGRESSION
- New Tier 2: Rotation and Tier 2: Carry exercise
- Progress to Jumping Pull-Up

Target Area: Mobility
Floor Medicine Ball Thoracic Rotations - 3 sets of 12 reps per side
Prisoner Frog Squat - 3 sets of 12 reps

Target Area: Core Stability
Push-Up Plank with Alternate Arm Raise - 3 sets of 12 reps per arm
Alternate Leg Raise Circles - 3 sets of 6 reps per leg, per direction

Tier 2: Rotation
Standing Cable Chop - 2 sets of 8 reps per side

Tier 1: Pull-Up
Jumping Pull-Up - 3 sets of 5 reps

Tier 2: Carry
Dumbbell Single Arm Farmer Walk - 3 sets of 30 yards each direction

Tier 2: Lunge
Dumbbell Goblet Reverse Lunge - 2 sets of 12 reps per leg

Target Area: Shoulder
Band Pull-Aparts - 3 sets of 15 reps

FRESHMAN/JV LEVEL   ALL SEASONAL

WEEK 4
Foundation Workout #12

WORKOUT PROGRESSION

- Taller box for Depth Drop
- Consider going for your Goblet Squat Test

Target Area: Mobility
PVC Bench Thoracic Extension - 3 sets of 30–45 seconds
Foam Roll Latissimus Dorsi (Lat) Muscles - 3 sets of 30 seconds each side

Target Area: Core Stability
Side Plank Inside Leg Raise - 3 sets of 8 reps
Renegade Row - 3 sets of 8 reps

Tier 2: Jump
Depth Drop Off Box (taller than last week) - 2 sets of 8 reps

Tier 1: Squat
Dumbbell Goblet Squat Test - 3 sets of 20 reps at 50% of your body weight

Tier 1: Chin-Up
Chin-Up Negatives (Eccentric) - 2 sets of 6 reps (1 rep = 3–5 second negative)

Tier 3: Posterior Chain
Try Glute Ham Raise - 2 sets of 8 reps
If not, try Slider Leg Curl or 45-degree Bench Back Extension - 2 sets of 20 reps

Target Area: Forearm
Barbell Wrist Curl - 2 sets of 10 reps

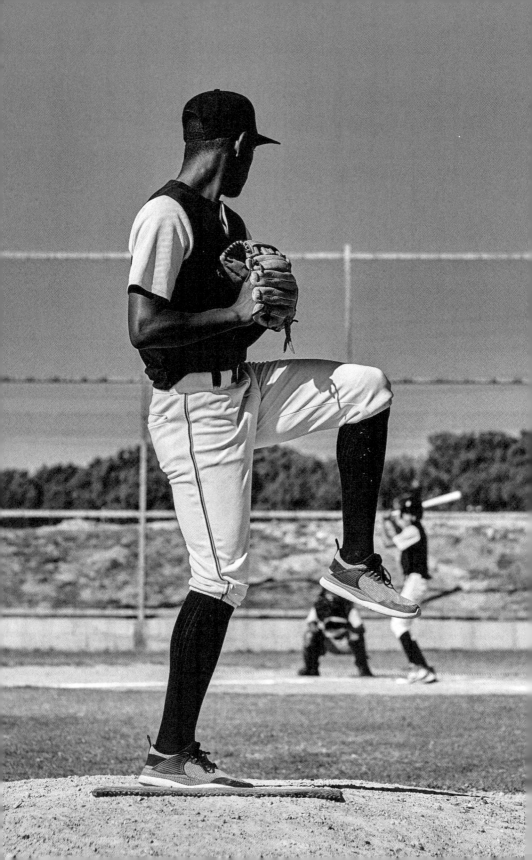

VARSITY LEVEL

IN-SEASON: SPRING

deally, we'd expect all varsity level athletes to train twice per week using a total body program. However, what a strength coach expects rarely matches up with what actually happens! Competing in 2–3 games per week, not to mention the logistics of the spring season—rain outs and game being rescheduled—can lead to inconsistent workouts in the weight room.

To resolve this, we build active recovery workouts that focus on core stability, shoulder prehab, forearm strength, and full body mobility exercises during the weeks students play three games. We also program strength exercise into team field warm-ups. Push-Ups, mini band lateral walks, single leg hops and jumps, and most medicine ball exercises can be done in the outfield.

The workouts in this section are smaller versions (fewer reps, sets, and training sessions) of their pre-season regimen to ensure complete recovery for games and important practices.

The starting pitchers will have a different routine based on game days, long toss, and bullpens days.

Program Breakdown: Position Player In-Season

Monday: Full Body	Wednesday: Full Body
Target Area: Mobility/Activation I & II Hip/Thoracic Mobility Glute Activation	**Target Area: Mobility/Activation I & II** Shoulder Mobility Upper Back Activation
Shoulder Prehab	**Shoulder Prehab**
"Big 5" Strength Deadlift	**"Big 5" Strength** Bench Press
Full Body Assistance I & II Shoulder Press Lunge	**Full Body Assistance I & II** Row or Pull-Up/Chin-Up Leg Curl
Forearm Strength	**Forearm Strength**

PROGRAM NOTES

- If pressed for time, you can super set the mobility/activation and assistance exercises as needed.

- Make minimal changes to the workout to prevent soreness in-season and to create a sense of routine.

- This program institutes exercise substitutions every three weeks to prevent plateaus and to keep the athletes mentally fresh.

- For the last few weeks of the season leading into post season play, the in-season program may simply consist of the mobility, activation, and prehab exercises.

- **Final note on in-season lifting:** It must be stressed that *everything* you do in the weight room must be geared towards keeping the athlete strong and injury-free late into the season. Make adjustments as needed.

PITCHER IN-SEASON PROGRAM OVERVIEW

This will obviously need to be adjusted to your situation; a high school pitcher may pitch more or less if the team has multiple starters, or if he plays another position while not pitching. Therefore, you may have to follow principles more so than during an in-season program.

The goal of the in-season pitcher program is two full body lifts between starts. One full body lift with a lower body strength emphasis is best the day after a start to allow for complete recovery before his next start. The second full body lift (with an upper body strength emphasis) is best after your bullpen (or long toss) session. A third optional lift of strictly power exercises consisting of medicine ball and jumps exercises (done in the outfield) is also a great option for weeks when a starter has more time between starts.

Try not to overthink this: one lift after a start and another lift after a bullpen session that week.

Point of emphasis: recall the section on Shoulder Prehab and Arm Care and use a slow and controlled tempo on all exercises for all reps.

After a Start Day	After a Bullpen Session
Target Area: Mobility/Activation I & II Hip/Thoracic Mobility Glute Activation	**Target Area: Mobility/Activation I & II** Shoulder Mobility Upper Back Activation
Shoulder Program	**Shoulder Program**
"Big 5" Lower Body Strength Deadlift or Box Squat	**Upper Pull Strength** Row or Pull-Up/Chin-Up
Full Body Assistance I & II Row Lunge	**Full Body Assistance I & II** Push-Up variation Leg Curl
Conditioning Long Sprints	**Conditioning** Short Sprints

VARSITY LEVEL   IN-SEASON: SPRING

GAME WEEK 1
Workout #1

Target Area: Mobility/Activation I
Single Leg Glute Bridge - 2–3 sets of 10–15 reps

Target Area: Mobility/Activation II
Lunge Yoga Rotations - 2–3 sets of 10–15 reps

Shoulder Prehab
Band Pull-Aparts - 3 sets of 25 reps

"Big 5" Strength
Trap Bar Deadlift - 3 sets of 5 reps at 80–85% max

Full Body Assistance I
Dumbbell Shoulder Press - 3 sets of 8 reps

Full Body Assistance II
Dumbbell Reverse Lunge - 3 sets of 8 reps per leg

Forearm Strength
1A. Dumbbell Wrist Extension - 3 sets of 12 reps
1B. Barbell Wrist Curl - 3 sets of 12 reps

GAME WEEK 1
Workout #2

Target Area: Mobility/Activation I
Yoga Push-Up - 2–3 sets of 10–15 reps

Target Area: Mobility/Activation II
Band Pull-Aparts - 2–3 sets of 25 reps

Shoulder Prehab
Bench Supported Dumbbell "Y" Raise - 3 sets of 15 reps

"Big 5" Strength
Dumbbell Bench Press - 3 sets of 5 reps at 80–85% max

Full Body Assistance I
Chin-Up/Pull-Up - 3 sets of 12 reps
Add Fat Gripz or a towel(s) for added forearm strength.

Full Body Assistance II
Glute Ham Raise - 3 sets of 12 reps

Forearm Strength
Build into Chin-up/Pull-up sets

VARSITY LEVEL   IN-SEASON: SPRING

GAME WEEK 2
Workout #1

WORKOUT NOTES

- "Big 5" strength exercise progressed to 85–90%

Target Area: Mobility/Activation I
Single Leg Glute Bridge - 2–3 sets of 10–15 reps

Target Area: Mobility/Activation II
Lunge Yoga Rotations - 2–3 sets of 10–15 reps

Shoulder Prehab
Band Pull-Aparts - 3 sets of 25 reps

"Big 5" Strength
Trap Bar Deadlift - 3 sets of 3 reps at 85–90% max

Full Body Assistance I
Dumbbell Shoulder Press - 3 sets of 8 reps

Full Body Assistance II
Dumbbell Reverse Lunge - 3 sets of 8 reps per leg

Forearm Strength
1A. Dumbbell Wrist Extension - 3 sets of 12 reps
1B. Barbell Wrist Curl - 3 sets of 12 reps

GAME WEEK 2
Workout #2

WORKOUT NOTES

- "Big 5" strength exercise progressed to 85–90%

Target Area: Mobility/Activation I
Yoga Push-Up - 2–3 sets of 10–15 reps

Target Area: Mobility/Activation II
Band Pull-Aparts - 2–3 sets of 25 reps

Shoulder Prehab
Bench Supported Dumbbell "Y" Raise - 3 sets of 15 reps

"Big 5" Strength
Dumbbell Bench Press - 3 sets of 3 reps at 85–90% of max

Full Body Assistance I
Chin-Up/Pull-Up - 3 sets of 12 reps
Add Fat Gripz or a towel(s) for added forearm strength.

Full Body Assistance II
Glute Ham Raise - 3 sets of 12 reps

Forearm Strength
Build into Chin-up/Pull-up sets

IN-SEASON: SPRING

VARSITY LEVEL

GAME WEEK 3
Workout #1

WORKOUT NOTES

- "Big 5" strength exercise pulled back to 75%

Target Area: Mobility/Activation I
Single Leg Glute Bridge - 2–3 sets of 10–15 reps

Target Area: Mobility/Activation II
Lunge Yoga Rotations - 2–3 sets of 10–15 reps

Shoulder Prehab
Band Pull-Aparts - 3 sets of 25 reps

"Big 5" Strength
Trap Bar Deadlift - 3 sets of 6 reps at 75% of max

Full Body Assistance I
Dumbbell Shoulder Press - 3 sets of 8 reps

Full Body Assistance II
Dumbbell Reverse Lunge - 3 sets of 8 reps per leg

Forearm Strength
1A. Dumbbell Wrist Extension - 3 sets of 12 reps
1B. Barbell Wrist Curl - 3 sets of 12 reps

GAME WEEK 3
Workout #2

WORKOUT NOTES

- "Big 5" strength exercise pulled back to 75% of max

Target Area: Mobility/Activation I
Yoga Push-Up - 2–3 sets of 10–15 reps

Target Area: Mobility/Activation II
Band Pull-Aparts - 2–3 sets of 25 reps

Shoulder Prehab
Bench Supported Dumbbell "Y" Raise - 3 sets of 15 reps

"Big 5" Strength
Dumbbell Bench Press - 3 sets of 6 reps at 75% of max

Full Body Assistance I
Chin-Up/Pull-Up - 3 sets of 12 reps
Add Fat Gripz or a towel(s) for added forearm strength.

Full Body Assistance II
Glute Ham Raise - 3 sets of 12 reps

Forearm Strength
Build into Chin-up/Pull-up sets

VARSITY LEVEL   IN-SEASON: SPRING

GAME WEEK 4
Workout #1

WORKOUT NOTES

- New "Big 5" strength exercise variation

Target Area: Mobility/Activation I
Single Leg Glute Bridge - 2–3 sets of 10–15 reps

Target Area: Mobility/Activation II
Lunge Yoga Rotations - 2–3 sets of 10–15 reps

Shoulder Prehab
Band Pull-Aparts - 3 sets of 25 reps

"Big 5" Strength
Barbell or Kettlebell Sumo Deadlift - 3 sets of 5 reps at 80–85% of your max

Full Body Assistance I
Dumbbell Shoulder Press - 3 sets of 8 reps

Full Body Assistance II
Dumbbell Reverse Lunge - 3 sets of 8 reps per leg

Forearm Strength
1A. Dumbbell Wrist Extension - 3 sets of 12 reps
1B. Barbell Wrist Curl - 3 sets of 12 reps

GAME WEEK 4
Workout #2

WORKOUT NOTES

- New "Big 5" strength exercise variation

Target Area: Mobility/Activation I
Yoga Push-Up - 2–3 sets of 10–15 reps

Target Area: Mobility/Activation II
Band Pull-Aparts - 2–3 sets of 25 reps

Shoulder Prehab
Bench Supported Dumbbell "Y" Raise - 3 sets of 15 reps

"Big 5" Strength
Dumbbell Incline Alternate Bench Press - 3 sets of 8 reps each arm

Full Body Assistance I
Chin-Up/Pull-Up - 3 sets of 12 reps
Add Fat Gripz or a towel(s) for added forearm strength.

Full Body Assistance II
Glute Ham Raise - 3 sets of 12 reps

Forearm Strength
Build into Chin-up/Pull-up sets

GAME WEEK 5
Workout #1

WORKOUT NOTES

- New mobility, shoulder prehab, forearm, and shoulder press exercises
- New "Big 5" strength exercise variation progressed to 85–90%

Target Area: Mobility/Activation I
Double Mini Band Squat - 3 sets of 20 reps
Position bands one above the knees, one below the knees.

Target Area: Mobility/Activation II
Lunge Yoga Rotations - 2–3 sets of 10–15 reps

Shoulder Prehab
Band or Cable Face Pull - 3 sets of 15 reps

"Big 5" Strength
Barbell or Kettlebell Sumo Deadlift - 3 sets of 3 reps at 85–90% of max

Full Body Assistance I
Dumbbell Single Arm Shoulder Press - 2 sets of 8 reps per arm

Full Body Assistance II
Dumbbell Reverse Lunge - 3 sets of 8 reps per leg

Forearm Strength
Wrist Roller – 2 sets of 2–3 reps (up and down = 1 rep)

GAME WEEK 5
Workout #2

WORKOUT NOTES

- New mobility, assistance, and forearm exercises

Target Area: Mobility/Activation I
Yoga Push-Up - 2–3 sets of 10–15 reps

Target Area: Mobility/Activation II
Walking Lunges with Overhead Reach - 2–3 sets of 12 each leg

Shoulder Prehab
Prone Prisoners - 3 sets of 8 reps (3 lbs. max)

"Big 5" Strength
Dumbbell Incline Alternate Bench Press - 3 sets of 8 reps each arm

Full Body Assistance I
TRX or Ring Row - 3 sets of 12–15 reps
Add Fat Gripz to the TRX Row or a towel(s) to the Ring Row for added forearm
   strength.

Full Body Assistance II
Physioball or Slider Leg Curl - 3 sets of 12 reps

Forearm Strength
Build into TRX or Ring Row sets

GAME WEEK 6
Workout #1

WORKOUT NOTES

- "Big 5" strength exercise pulled back to 75% of max

Target Area: Mobility/Activation I
Double Mini Band Squat - 3 sets of 20 reps
Position bands one above the knees, one below the knees

Target Area: Mobility/Activation II
Lunge Yoga Rotations - 2–3 sets of 10–15 reps

Shoulder Prehab
Band or Cable Face Pull - 3 sets of 15 reps

"Big 5" Strength
Barbell or Kettlebell Sumo Deadlift - 3 sets of 6 reps at 75% of max

Full Body Assistance I
Dumbbell Single Arm Shoulder Press - 2 sets of 8 reps per arm

Full Body Assistance II
Dumbbell Reverse Lunge - 3 sets of 8 reps per leg

Forearm Strength
Wrist Roller – 2 sets of 2–3 reps (up and down = 1 rep)

GAME WEEK 6
Workout #2

WORKOUT NOTES

- Volume increased on dumbbell incline bench press
- Substitute Battle Rope Row for TRX or Ring Row if possible. Simply loop a Battle Rope (2 inch thick ropes are best) over your power rack for the best set-up.

Target Area: Mobility/Activation I
Yoga Push-Up - 2–3 sets of 10–15 reps

Target Area: Mobility/Activation II
Walking Lunges with Overhead Reach - 2–3 sets of 12 each leg

Shoulder Prehab
Prone Prisoners - 3 sets of 8 reps (3 lbs. max)

"Big 5" Strength
Dumbbell Incline Alternate Bench Press - 4 sets of 6 reps each arm

Full Body Assistance I
TRX or Ring Row - 3 sets of 12–15 reps
Add Fat Gripz to the TRX Row or a towel(s) to the Ring Row for added forearm
    strength.

Full Body Assistance II
Physioball or Slider Leg Curl - 3 sets of 12 reps

Forearm Strength
Build into TRX or Ring Row sets

IN-SEASON: SPRING   VARSITY LEVEL

GAME WEEK 7
Workout #1

WORKOUT NOTES

- Return to "Big 5" strength exercises of Weeks 1, 2, and 3 with decreased volume for the final weeks of the season.

Target Area: Mobility/Activation I
Double Mini Band Squat - 3 sets of 20 reps
Position bands one above the knees, one below the knees

Target Area: Mobility/Activation II
Lunge Yoga Rotations - 2–3 sets of 10–15 reps

Shoulder Prehab
Band or Cable Face Pull - 3 sets of 15 reps

"Big 5" Strength
Trap Bar Deadlift - 3 sets of 3 reps at 80–85% of max

Full Body Assistance I
Dumbbell Single Arm Shoulder Press - 2 sets of 8 reps per arm

Full Body Assistance II
Dumbbell Reverse Lunge - 3 sets of 8 reps per leg

Forearm Strength
Wrist Roller - 2 sets of 2–3 reps (up and down = 1 rep)

GAME WEEK 7
Workout #2

WORKOUT NOTES

- Return to "Big 5" strength exercises of Weeks 1, 2, and 3 with decreased volume for the final weeks of the season.
- Substitute Battle Rope Row for TRX or Ring Row if possible. Simply loop a Battle Rope (2 inch thick ropes are best) over your power rack for the best set-up.

Target Area: Mobility/Activation I
Yoga Push-Up - 2–3 sets of 10–15 reps

Target Area: Mobility/Activation II
Walking Lunges with Overhead Reach - 2–3 sets of 12 each leg

Shoulder Prehab
Prone Prisoners - 3 sets of 8 reps (3 lbs. MAX)

"Big 5" Strength
Dumbbell Bench Press - 3 sets of 3 reps at 80–85% of max
Optional Push-ups - 2 sets of 15-25 reps

Full Body Assistance I
TRX or Ring Row - 3 sets of 12–15 reps
Add Fat Gripz to the TRX Row or a towel(s) to the Ring Row for added forearm
    strength.

Full Body Assistance II
Physioball or Slider Leg Curl - 3 sets of 12 reps

Forearm Strength
Build into TRX or Ring Row sets

GAME WEEK 8
Workout #1

WORKOUT NOTES

- "Big 5" strength exercise decreased in volume and intensity to accommodate the grueling season.

Target Area: Mobility/Activation I
Double Mini Band Squat - 3 sets of 20 reps
Position bands one above the knees, one below the knees

Target Area: Mobility/Activation II
Lunge Yoga Rotations - 2–3 sets of 10–15 reps

Shoulder Prehab
Band or Cable Face Pull - 3 sets of 15 reps

"Big 5" Strength
Trap Bar Deadlift - 2 sets of 3 reps at 75–80% of max

Full Body Assistance I
Dumbbell Single Arm Shoulder Press - 2 sets of 8 reps per arm

Full Body Assistance II
Dumbbell Reverse Lunge - 3 sets of 8 reps per leg

Forearm Strength
Wrist Roller - 2 sets of 2–3 reps (up and down = 1 rep)

GAME WEEK 8
Workout #2

WORKOUT NOTES

- "Big 5" strength exercise decreased in volume and intensity to accommodate the grueling season.
- Substitute Battle Rope Row for TRX or Ring Row if possible. Simply loop a Battle Rope (2 inch thick ropes are best) over your power rack for the best set-up.

Target Area: Mobility/Activation I
Yoga Push-Up - 2–3 sets of 10–15 reps

Target Area: Mobility/Activation II
Walking Lunges with Overhead Reach - 2–3 sets of 12 each leg

Shoulder Prehab
Prone Prisoners - 3 sets of 5-8 reps (3 lbs. max)

"Big 5" Strength
Dumbbell Bench Press - 2 sets of 3 reps at 75–80% of max
Optional Push-ups – 2 sets of 15-25 reps

Full Body Assistance I
TRX or Ring Row - 3 sets of 12–15 reps
Add Fat Gripz to the TRX Row or a towel(s) to the Ring Row for added forearm strength

Full Body Assistance II
Physioball or Slider Leg Curl - 3 sets of 12 reps

Forearm Strength
Build into TRX or Ring Row sets

IN-SEASON: SPRING   VARSITY LEVEL

GAME WEEK (PITCHERS)
Workout #1

WORKOUT NOTES

- Pitchers do the same workout all season long to prevent soreness. Please adjust volume (reps and sets) as needed.
- I give my Varsity pitchers the option of Deadlift or Squat.
- The YOKE Bar is an amazing tool if you have access. The bar allows the shoulders to be in a comfortable, neutral position during heavy squat movements.

Target Area: Mobility/Activation I
Single Leg Glute Bridge - 2–3 sets of 10–15 reps

Target Area: Mobility/Activation II
Lunge Yoga Rotations - 2–3 sets of 10–15 reps

Shoulder Program
1A. Band Pull-Aparts - 3 sets of 25 reps
1B. Bench Supported External Rotations - 3 sets of 12

"Big 5" Strength
Trap Bar Deadlift - 3 sets of 5 reps at 80–85% max
    OR
YOKE Bar Box Squat - 3 sets of 5 reps at 80–85% max

Full Body Assistance I
TRX or Ring Row - 3 sets of 12–15 reps
Optional: Add Fat Gripz to the TRX Row or a towel(s) to the Ring Row for added forearm strength.

Full Body Assistance II
Dumbbell Reverse Lunge - 3 sets of 8 reps per leg

Conditioning Option #1: Sprints
Run 8–12 30-yard sprints
Recover during the walk back to the starting line.

Conditioning Option #2: Medicine Ball Circuit

1A. Medicine Ball Squat and Press Throw - 3 sets of 5 throws
>Holding a medicine ball at your chin, quickly squat down, jump up and throw the medicine ball in the air. Allow the ball to hit ground. Do not catch.

1B. Medicine Ball Reverse Scoop Throw - 3 sets of 4 throws (2 each direction)
>Holding a medicine ball at your waist, quickly deadlift/hinge down, jump up, and throw the medicine ball backward over your head in the air. Jog to the ball and throw it back.

1C. Medicine Ball (MB) Power Exercise III
>Holding a medicine ball at your waist, jump laterally (sideways) to your right, decelerate by landing on the outside leg, then jump the opposite direction, laterally (sideways) to your left and throw the medicine ball for distance. Jog to the ball and throw it back.

1D. Medicine Ball Lateral Bound Rotation Throws
>Bound (jump) from your left to your right foot, change directions, and throw the medicine ball to the left for distance.

GAME WEEK (PITCHERS)
Workout #2

WORKOUT NOTES

- Pitchers do the same workout all season to prevent soreness. Please adjust volume (reps and sets) as needed.
- I give my varsity pitchers the option of Row or Pull-Up/Chin-Up. Typically, the bigger pitchers do Rows and the smaller pitchers do pull ups.

Target Area: Mobility/Activation I
Yoga Push-Up - 2–3 sets of 10–15 reps

Target Area: Mobility/Activation II
Band Pull-Aparts - 2–3 sets of 25 reps

Shoulder Program
1A. Bench Supported Dumbbell "Y" Raise - 3 sets of 15 reps
1B. Cable or Band Face Pull - 3 sets of 15 reps

"Big 5" Strength
Row or Pull-Up/Chin-Up based on strength level - 3 sets of 8–12 reps
Optional: add Fat Gripz to the TRX Row or a towel(s) to the Ring Row for added forearm strength.

Full Body Assistance I
Push-up variation - 3 sets of 10-25 reps based on strength level

Full Body Assistance II
Glute Ham Raise - 3 sets of 12 reps

Conditioning Option #1 - Sprints
Run 10–15 10-yard sprints
Recover during the walk back to the starting line.

Conditioning Option #2: Medicine Ball Circuit

1A. Medicine Ball Squat and Press Throw - 3 sets of 5 throws
Holding a medicine ball at your chin, quickly squat down, jump up, and throw the medicine ball in the air. Allow the ball to hit ground. Do not catch.

1B. Medicine Ball Reverse Scoop Throw - 3 sets of 4 throws (2 each direction)
Holding a medicine ball at your waist, quickly deadlift/hinge down, jump up, and throw the medicine ball backward over your head in the air. Jog to the ball and throw it back.

1C. Medicine Ball (MB) Power Exercise III
Holding a medicine ball at your waist, jump laterally (sideways) to your right, decelerate by landing on the outside leg, then jump the opposite direction, laterally (sideways) to your left and throw the medicine ball for distance. Jog to the ball and throw it back.

1D. Medicine Ball Lateral Bound Rotation Throws
Bound (jump) from your left to your right foot, change directions, and throw the medicine ball to the left for distance.

GAME WEEK (PITCHERS)
Optional Power Workout #3

WORKOUT NOTES

- This medicine ball based workout can be done in the outfield.
- Allow for full rest between sets. The workout is designed to last 20 minutes, start to finish.

Target Area: Mobility/Activation I
Double Mini Band Squat - 3 sets of 20 reps
Position bands one above the knees, one below the knees.

Target Area: Mobility/Activation II
Walking Lunges with Overhead Reach - 2–3 sets of 12 each leg

Shoulder Prehab
Prone Prisoners - 3 sets of 8 reps (3 lbs. max)

Medicine Ball Power Exercise I
Medicine Ball Squat and Press Throw - 3 sets of 5 throws
Holding a medicine ball at your chin, quickly squat down, jump up, and throw the medicine ball in the air. Allow the ball to hit ground. Do not catch.

Medicine Ball Power Exercise II
Medicine Ball Reverse Scoop Throw - 3 sets of 4 throws (2 each direction)
Holding a medicine ball at your waist, quickly deadlift/hinge down, jump up, and throw the medicine ball backward over your head in the air. Jog to the ball and throw it back.

Medicine Ball Power Exercise III
Medicine Ball Lateral Bound and Rotation Throw - 3 sets of 4 throws (2 each direction)
Holding a medicine ball at your waist, jump laterally (sideways) to your right, decelerate by landing on the outside leg, then jump the opposite direction, laterally (sideways) to your left and throw the medicine ball for distance. Jog to the ball and throw it back.

POST-SEASON I (LATE SPRING/EARLY SUMMER)

During this 4-week GPP (general physical preparation) phase, we program for some variations on the "Big 5," focusing on rebuilding stability and developing a solid range of motion after a grueling season. We do not do sprint or dynamic work (jumping or medicine ball work) and minimize loads on the barbell to allow for further recovery. The focus during this phase is low intensity prehab, mobility, core stability, body weight strength, and massage work.

This is also when most travel programs start up, and kids may be reluctant to get in the weight room. Even worse, they may be discouraged by ignorant head baseball coaches. If you want to play in college—if you want to be the best—then remember that the sign of a champion is someone who does the work when no one is watching!

Program Breakdown

Daily Workout

Prehab Warm-Up
Upper Back Activation
Hip and Thoracic Mobility

Target Area: Front Squat Mobility
Wrist
Thoracic Extension

Target Area: Core Stability
Anterior Stability
Lateral Stability

"Big 5" Dumbbell Variation
Day 1: Dumbbell Goblet Squat
Day 2: Dumbbell Bench Press
Day 3: Dumbbell RDL

Tier 1: Body Weight Strength
Lower Body
Upper Body

Recovery: Foam Roll Massage

PROGRAM NOTES

- Do each set of workouts for 2 weeks. Players who did not play as much during the active season can push more weight in this phase.

- This is a great time to involve the freshman and JV players because the movements are less technical.

WEEK 1
Workout #1

Prehab Warm-Up
Band Pull-Aparts - 3 sets of 25 reps
Walking Lunge with Rotation - 3 sets of 12 reps per leg

Target Area: Front Squat Mobility
Bench Wrist Stretch - 3 sets for 30–45 seconds each
    Rotate your hands so your fingers are facing you and place hands on a bench.
PVC Bench Thoracic Extension - 3 sets for 30–45 seconds each

Target Area: Core Stability
Physioball Front Plank Circles - 3 sets of 30–45 seconds
Alternate Leg Raise - 3 sets of 10 reps per leg

"Big 5" Variation
Dumbbell Goblet Squat - 12, 10, 8, 6

Tier 1: Body Weight Strength
TRX Leg Curl - 3 sets of 15 reps
Floor, TRX, or Ring Push-Up - 3 sets of 15–25 reps

Foam Roll Massage
3–5 minutes of IT bands, calves, quads, and upper back

WEEK 1
Workout #2

Prehab Warm-Up
Dumbbell "T" Raise - 3 sets of 15 reps
Single Leg Glute Bridge - 3 sets of 12 reps per leg

Target Area: Front Squat Mobility
Foam Roll Latissimus Dorsi (Lat) Muscles - 3 sets of 20 rolls
Medicine Ball Thoracic Extension - 3 sets of 6 deep breaths

Target Area: Core Stability
Physioball Dead Bug - 3 sets of 8 reps (slow)
Side Plank - 3 sets of 45 seconds per side

"Big 5" Variations
Dumbbell Bench Press - 12, 10, 8, 6, 12

Tier 1: Body Weight Strength
TRX Row or Chin-Up - 3 sets of 8–12 reps
Bulgarian Squat - 3 sets of 15 reps per leg

Foam Roll Massage
3–5 minutes on IT bands, calves, quads, and upper back

WEEK 1
Workout #3

Prehab Warm-Up
Dumbbell "T" Balance - 3 sets of 8 reps per leg
PVC Overhead Squat (heels elevated) - 3 sets of 15 reps

Target Area: Front Squat Mobility
Bench Wrist Stretch - 3 sets for 30–45 seconds
> Rotate your hands so your fingers are facing you and place hands on a bench.

Kneeling Thoracic Rotations - 3 sets of 6 deep breaths each side
> Rest your glutes on your heels while kneeling. Place your fist on your temple and rotate your elbow to the sky.

Target Area: Core Stability
Push-Up Plank with Alternate Arm Raised - 3 sets of 12 reps per arm
Alternate Leg Raise Circles - 3 sets of 6 reps per leg in each direction

"Big 5" Variations
Dumbbell RDL - 12, 10, 8, 6

Tier 1: Body Weight Strength
Pause Stationary Lateral Lunge - 3 sets of 6 reps per leg (3 second pause per rep)
Pulldown or Seated Row Machine - 3 sets of 12 reps

Foam Roll Massage
3–5 minutes on IT bands, calves, quads, and upper back

WEEK 2
Workout #1

Prehab Warm-Up
Band Pull-Aparts - 3 sets of 25 reps
Walking Lunge with Rotation - 3 sets of 12 reps per leg

Target Area: Front Squat Mobility
Bench Wrist Stretch - 3 sets for 30–45 seconds
    Rotate your hands so your fingers are facing you and place your hands on a
        bench
PVC Bench Thoracic Extension - 3 sets for 30–45 seconds

Target Area: Core Stability
Physioball Front Plank Circles - 3 sets for 30–45 seconds
Alternate Leg Raise - 3 sets of 10 reps per leg

"Big 5" Variation
Dumbbell Goblet Squat - 12, 10, 8, 6

Tier 1: Body Weight Strength
TRX Leg Curl - 3 sets of 15 reps
Floor, TRX, or Ring Push-Up - 3 sets for 15–25 seconds

Foam Roll Massage
3–5 minutes on IT bands, calves, quads, and upper back

WEEK 2
Workout #2

POST-SEASON I (LATE SPRING/EARLY SUMMER)

VARSITY LEVEL

Prehab Warm-Up
Dumbbell "T" Raise - 3 sets of 15 reps
Single Leg Glute Bridge - 3 sets of 12 reps per leg

Target Area: Front Squat Mobility
Foam Roll Latissimus Dorsi (Lat) Muscles - 3 sets of 20 rolls
Medicine Ball Thoracic Extension - 3 sets of 6 deep breaths

Target Area: Core Stability
Physioball Dead Bug - 3 sets of 8 reps (slow)
Side Plank - 3 sets for 45 seconds per side

"Big 5" Variations
Dumbbell Bench Press - 12, 10, 8, 6, 12

Tier 1: Body Weight Strength
TRX Row or Chin-Up - 3 sets of 8–12 reps
Bulgarian Squat - 3 sets of 15 reps per leg

Foam Roll Massage
3–5 minutes on IT bands, calves, quads, and upper back

WEEK 2
Workout #3

Prehab Warm-Up
Dumbbell "T" Balance - 3 sets of 8 reps per leg
PVC Overhead Squat (heels elevated) - 3 sets of 15 reps

Target Area: Front Squat Mobility
Bench Wrist Stretch - 3 sets for 30–45 seconds
    Rotate your hands so your fingers are facing you and place them on a bench
Kneeling Thoracic Rotations - 3 sets of 6 deep breaths per side
    Rest your glutes on your heels while kneeling. Place your fist on your temple
        and rotate your elbow to the sky.

Target Area: Core Stability
Push-Up Plank with Alternate Arm Raise - 3 sets of 12 reps per arm
Alternate Leg Raise Circles - 3 sets of 6 reps per leg in each direction

"Big 5" Variations
Dumbbell RDL - 12, 10, 8, 6

Tier 1: Body Weight Strength
Pause Stationary Lateral Lunge - 3 sets of 6 reps per leg (3 second pause per
    rep)
Pulldown or Seated Row Machine - 3 sets of 12 reps

Foam Roll Massage
3–5 minutes on IT bands, calves, quads, and upper back

POST-SEASON II (LATE SPRING/EARLY SUMMER)

During these two weeks, we focus on additional thoracic mobility to better prepare for front squats in the coming months. Front squat mobility becomes front squat technique; this is likely the first time many of your players will put a barbell on their shoulders. The dumbbell goblet squat now has additional volume and, for variation, the dumbbell bench incline press and glute bridge are programmed. Finally, new body weight strength exercises are added.

Program Breakdown

Daily Workout
Prehab Warm-Up
Upper Back Activation
Hip Mobility
Thoracic Spine Mobility
Tier 1: Front Squat (Technique)
Frankenstein or Lifting Strap Front Squat
Target Area: Core Stability
Anterior Stability
Lateral Stability
"Big 5" Dumbbell Variation
Day 1: Dumbbell Goblet Squat
Day 2: Dumbbell Bench Incline Press
Day 3: Dumbbell Glute Bridge
Tier 1: Body Weight Strength
Lower Body
Upper Body
Foam Roll Massage

PROGRAM NOTES

- Do each set of workouts for 2 weeks. Those who did not play as much during active season can push more weight in this phase.
- This is a great time to involve the freshman and JV players because the movements are less technical.

WEEK 3
Workout #1

WORKOUT PROGRESSIONS

- More volume for dumbbell goblet squats
- New body weight exercises
- Reintroduction of front squat technique exercises for varsity players
- Additional thoracic mobility exercise to the prehab warm up

Prehab Warm-Up
Band Pull-Aparts - 3 sets of 25 reps
Walking Lunge with Rotation - 3 sets of 12 reps per leg
Medicine Ball Thoracic Extension - 3 sets of 6 deep breaths

Tier 1: Front Squat (Technique)
Frankenstein Front Squat (empty barbell) - 3 sets of 12 reps

Target Area: Core Stability
Physioball Front Plank Circles - 3 sets for 30–45 seconds
Alternate Leg Raise - 3 sets of 10 reps each leg

"Big 5" Variation
Dumbbell Goblet Squat - 3 sets of 15–25 reps

Tier 1: Body Weight Strength
TRX Glute Bridge - 3 sets of 15 reps
Floor, TRX, or Ring Push-Up - 3 sets of 15–25 reps (feet elevated)

Foam Roll Massage
3–5 minutes on IT bands, calves, quads, and upper back

WEEK 3
Workout #2

POST-SEASON II (LATE SPRING/EARLY SUMMER)

VARSITY LEVEL

WORKOUT PROGRESSIONS

- New "Big 5" exercise variations
- New body weight exercise and progression to dumbbells
- Reintroduction of front squat technique exercises for varsity players
- Additional thoracic mobility exercise to the prehab warm up

Prehab Warm-Up
Dumbbell "T" Raise - 3 sets of 15 reps
Single Leg Glute Bridge - 3 sets of 12 reps per leg
PVC Bench Thoracic Extension - 3 sets for 30–45 seconds

Tier 1: Front Squat (Technique)
Frankenstein Front Squat (empty barbell) - 3 sets of 12 reps

Target Area: Core Stability
Physioball Dead Bug - 3 sets of 8 reps (slow)
Side Plank - 3 sets of 45 seconds per side

"Big 5" Variations
Dumbbell Incline Bench Press - 12, 10, 8, 6, 12

Tier 1: Body Weight Strength
TRX Row or Chin-Up - 3 sets of 12–15 reps
Dumbbell Goblet Bulgarian Squat - 3 sets of 15 reps per leg

Foam Roll Massage
3–5 minutes on IT bands, calves, quads, and upper back

WEEK 3
Workout #3

WORKOUT PROGRESSIONS

- New "Big 5" exercise variation
- New body weight exercises
- Reintroduction of front squat technique exercises for varsity players
- Additional thoracic mobility exercise to the prehab warm up

Prehab Warm-Up
Dumbbell "T" Balance - 3 sets of 8 reps per leg
PVC Overhead Squat (heels elevated) - 3 sets of 15 reps
Kneeling Thoracic Rotations - 3 sets of 6 deep breaths per side
> Rest your glutes on your heels while kneeling. Place your fist on your temple and rotate your elbow to the sky.

Tier 1: Front Squat (Technique)
Frankenstein Front Squat (empty barbell) - 3 sets of 12 reps

Target Area: Core Stability
Push-Up Plank with Alternate Arm Raise - 3 sets of 12 reps per arm
Alternate Leg Raise Circles - 3 sets of 6 reps per leg in each direction

"Big 5" Variations
Barbell Glute Bridge or Barbell Hip Thrust - 12, 10, 8, 6

Tier 1: Body Weight Strength
Lateral Squat - 3 sets of 12 reps per leg
> Shift laterally in a lateral lunge stance, maintaining your squat depth.
Dumbbell One-Arm Row - 3 sets of 8 reps per arm

Foam Roll Massage
3–5 minutes on IT bands, calves, quads, and upper back

WEEK 4
Workout #1

WORKOUT PROGRESSIONS

- Add weight to the dumbbell goblet squat

Prehab Warm-Up
Band Pull-Aparts - 3 sets of 25 reps
Walking Lunge with Rotation - 3 sets of 12 reps per leg
Medicine Ball Thoracic Extension - 3 sets of 6 deep breaths

Tier 1: Front Squat (Technique)
Frankenstein Front Squat (empty barbell) - 3 sets of 12 reps
    Add some light weight to the barbell if you feel confident after practicing with
        an empty barbell during the last three weeks.

Target Area: Core Stability
Physioball Front Plank Circles - 3 sets for 30–45 seconds
Alternate Leg Raise - 3 sets of 10 reps per leg

"Big 5" Variation
Dumbbell Goblet Squat - 3 sets of 15–25 reps

Tier 1: Body Weight Strength
TRX Glute Bridge - 3 sets of 15 reps
Floor, TRX, or Ring Push-Up - 3 sets of 15–25 reps (feet elevated)

Foam Roll Massage
3–5 minutes on IT bands, calves, quads, and upper back

WEEK 4
Workout #2

WORKOUT PROGRESSIONS

- Add weight to the dumbbell incline bench press

Prehab Warm-Up
Dumbbell "T" Raise - 3 sets of 15 reps
Single Leg Glute Bridge - 3 sets of 12 reps per leg
PVC Bench Thoracic Extension - 3 sets of 30–45 seconds

Tier 1: Front Squat (Technique)
Frankenstein Front Squat (empty barbell) - 3 sets of 12 reps
> Add some light weight to the barbell if you feel confident after practicing with an empty barbell during the last three weeks.

Target Area: Core Stability
Physioball Dead Bug - 3 sets of 8 super slow reps
Side Plank - 3 sets of 45 seconds per side

"Big 5" Variations
Dumbbell Incline Bench Press – 10, 8, 6, 10

Tier 1: Body Weight Strength
TRX Row or Chin-Up - 3 sets of 12–15 reps
Dumbbell Goblet Bulgarian Squat - 3 sets of 15 reps per leg

Foam Roll Massage
3–5 minutes on IT bands, calves, quads, and upper back

WEEK 4
Workout #3

WORKOUT PROGRESSIONS

- Add weight to the barbell glute bridge or hip thrust

Prehab Warm-Up
Dumbbell "T" Balance - 3 sets of 8 reps per leg
PVC Overhead Squat (heels elevated) - 3 sets of 15 reps
Kneeling Thoracic Rotations - 3 sets of 6 deep breaths per side
> Rest your glutes on your heels while kneeling. Place your fist on your temple and rotate your elbow to the sky.

Tier 1: Front Squat (Technique)
Frankenstein Front Squat (empty barbell) - 3 sets of 12 reps
> Add some light weight to the barbell if you feel confident after practicing with an empty barbell during the last three weeks.

Target Area: Core Stability
Push-Up Plank with Alternate Arm Raise - 3 sets of 12 reps per arm
Alternate Leg Raise Circles - 3 sets of 6 reps per leg in each direction

"Big 5" Variations
Barbell Glute Bridge or Barbell Hip Thrust - 12, 10, 8, 6

Tier 1: Body Weight Strength
Lateral Squat - 3 sets of 12 reps each leg
> Shift laterally in a lateral lunge stance, maintaining your squat depth.
Dumbbell One-Arm Row - 3 sets of 8 reps per arm

Foam Roll Massage
3–5 minutes on IT bands, calves, quads, and upper back

OFF-SEASON I (SUMMER)

C oming off the GPP phase and for the second half of the summer, we build on the "Big 5" with a focus on eccentric and isometric work while striving to build size and strength with four lift days per week: two upper body and two lower body. This is a seven-week program featuring six high intensity weeks separated by one recovery week in the middle. This offers a great opportunity to start building muscle mass. Those looking to drop body fat going into the next season can add non-impact cardio to burn extra calories unless they're playing an intense travel baseball schedule.

Note: During this phase, senior student athletes who have committed to play college baseball will follow a separate program—namely, the program sent to them by the college or university. The focus for these athletes will be learning what will be expected from them in a college weight room.

Program Breakdown

Monday	Tuesday	Thursday	Friday
Target Area: Mobility/Core Stability Warm-Up	**Target Area:** Mobility/Core Stability Warm-Up	**Target Area:** Mobility/Core Stability Warm-Up	**Target Area:** Mobility/Core Stability Warm-Up
Tier 2: Vertical Jump (Isometric)	**Tier 2:** Throw	**Tier 2:** Lateral Jump (Isometric)	**Tier 2:** Rotation
	Tier 1: Bench Press (Eccentric)		**Tier 1:** Pull-Up/ Chin-Up
Tier 1: Front Squat (Eccentric)		**Tier 1:** Trap Bar Deadlift (Eccentric)	
Tier 1: Deadlift	**Upper Body Assistance**		**Upper Body Assistance**
		Tier 1: Squat	
Tier 2: Lunge	**Tier 1:** Body Weight Strength	**Tier 2:** Lunge	**Tier 1:** Body Weight Strength
Tier 3: Glute Bridge		**Tier 3:** Leg Curl	
	Tier 2: Carry		**Tier 2:** Carry

PROGRAM NOTES

- This phase emphasizes building up one "Big 5" exercise each day.
- Continue practicing the skills of the front squat exercise from the previous off-season phase.
- Continue building volume for the body weight exercises from the previous off-season phase and progress the dumbbell and barbell versions.
- Assistance work in this phase focuses on Tier 2 and 3 core lift movements: carry, lunge, rotate, throw, glute bridge, leg curl, shoulder press, and row.

VARSITY LEVEL   OFF-SEASON I (SUMMER)

WEEK 1
Workout #1: Lower Body/Squat Day

WORKOUT NOTES

- Circuit the mobility and core stability warm-up and limit to 10 minutes.

Target Area: Mobility/Core Stability Warm-Up
Walking Lunge with Rotation - 3 sets of 12 reps per leg
Physioball Front Plank Circles - 3 sets for 30–45 seconds
Medicine Ball Thoracic Extension - 3 sets of 6 deep breaths
Alternate Leg Raise - 3 sets of 10 reps per leg

Tier 2: Vertical Jump (Isometric)
Squat Jump Isometric (stick and hold each landing for 2 seconds) - 3 sets of 5
  jumps

"Big 5" Strength
Barbell Front Box Squat (Eccentric)
Perform each rep with 3 seconds eccentric (slow and controlled movement
  down).
Set 1: 8 reps at 45% max weight
Set 2: 8 reps at 55% max weight
Set 3: 8 reps at 65% max weight
Set 4: 8 reps at 75% max weight

Tier 1: Deadlift
Barbell RDL - 3 sets of 10 reps

Tier 2: Lunge
Dumbbell Reverse Lunge - 3 sets of 10 reps per leg

Tier 3: Glute Bridge
Single Leg Glute Bridge - 3 sets of 10 reps per leg

WEEK 1
Workout #2: Upper Body/Bench Day

WORKOUT NOTES
- Circuit the mobility and core stability warm-up and limit to 10 minutes.

Target Area: Mobility/Core Stability Warm-Up
Dumbbell "T" Raise - 3 sets of 15 reps
Physioball Dead Bug - 3 sets of 8 super slow reps
PVC Bench Thoracic Extension - 3 sets for 30–45 seconds
Side Plank - 3 sets of 45 seconds per side

Tier 2: Throw
Medicine Ball Squat Press Throw - 3 sets of 5 reps

"Big 5" Strength
Dumbbell Bench Press (Eccentric)
Perform each rep with 3 seconds eccentric (slow and controlled movement
    down).
Set 1: 8 reps at 45% max weight
Set 2: 8 reps at 55% max weight
Set 3: 8 reps at 65% max weight
Set 4: 8 reps at 75% max weight

Upper Body Assistance
Barbell Row - 3 sets of 10 reps
Dumbbell Incline Chest Press - 3 sets of 10 reps

Tier 1: Body Weight Strength
TRX or Ring Row - 2 sets of 12 reps
Dumbbell Rear Delt Raise - 2 sets of 15 reps

Tier 2: Carry
Dumbbell or Trap Bar Farmer Walks - 3 sets of 40 yards

WEEK 1
Workout #3: Lower Body/Deadlift Day

WORKOUT NOTES
- Circuit the mobility and core stability warm-up and limit to 10 minutes.

Target Area: Mobility/Core Stability Warm-Up
Walking Lunge with Rotation - 3 sets of 12 reps per leg
Physioball Front Plank Circles - 3 sets for 30–45 seconds
Medicine Ball Thoracic Extension - 3 sets of 6 deep breaths
Alternate Leg Raise - 3 sets of 10 reps per leg

Tier 2: Lateral Jump (Isometric)
Lateral Squat Jump Isometric (stick and hold each landing for 2 seconds) - 3 sets
of 3 jumps in each direction

"Big 5" Strength
Trap Bar Deadlift (Eccentric)
Perform each rep with 3 seconds eccentric (slow and controlled movement
down).
Set 1: 8 reps at 45% max weight
Set 2: 8 reps at 55% max weight
Set 3: 8 reps at 65% max weight
Set 4: 8 reps at 75% max weight

Tier 1: Squat
Barbell Back Box Squat - 3 sets of 10 reps

Tier 2: Lunge
Dumbbell Lateral Lunge - 3 sets of 10 reps per leg

Leg Curl
Physioball Leg Curl - 2 sets of 12 reps

WEEK 1
Workout #4: Upper Body/Pull-Up Day

WORKOUT NOTES

- Circuit the mobility and core stability warm-up and limit to 10 minutes.
- If the athlete cannot perform a full pull-up or chin-up, please substitute their pull-up/chin-up progression exercise into the "Big 5" strength section.
- Do as few sets as possible to accumulate the total pull-up/chin-up reps of the week, max 10 reps per set. Add a weight vest or chain after the athlete has progressed past 3 sets of 10 reps of body weight reps.

Target Area: Mobility/Core Stability Warm-Up
Dumbbell "T" Raise - 3 sets of 15 reps
Physioball Dead Bug - 3 sets of 8 super slow reps
PVC Bench Thoracic Extension - 3 sets for 30–45 seconds
Side Plank - 3 sets of 45 seconds per side

Tier 2: Rotation
Cable Chop or Medicine Ball Rotational Throw - 3 sets of 8 reps

"Big 5" Strength
Pull-Up/Chin-Up (weights optional) - 25 reps in as few sets as possible (see
    Workout Notes above)

Upper Body Assistance
Dumbbell Shoulder Press - 3 sets of 10 reps
One-Arm Dumbbell Row - 3 sets of 10 reps per arm

Tier 1: Body Weight Strength
TRX or Ring Push-Up - 2 sets of 12 reps
Dumbbell Lateral Raise - 2 sets of 15 reps

Tier 2: Carry
Dumbbell or Trap Bar Farmer Walks - 3 sets of 40 yards

OFF-SEASON I (SUMMER)

VARSITY LEVEL

WEEK 2
Workout #1: Lower Body/Squat Day

WORKOUT NOTES

- Circuit the mobility and core stability warm-up and limit to 10 minutes.
- Consider adding weight to the RDL this week

Target Area: Mobility/Core Stability Warm-Up
Walking Lunge with Rotation - 3 sets of 12 reps per leg
Physioball Front Plank Circles - 3 sets for 30–45 seconds
Medicine Ball Thoracic Extension - 3 sets of 6 deep breaths
Alternate Leg Raise - 3 sets of 10 reps per leg

Tier 2: Vertical Jump (Isometric)
Squat Jump Isometric (stick and hold each landing for 2 seconds) - 3 sets of 5
jumps

"Big 5" Strength
Barbell Front Box Squat (Eccentric)
Perform each rep with 4 seconds eccentric (slow and controlled movement
down).
Set 1: 6 reps at 50% max weight
Set 2: 6 reps at 60% max weight
Set 3: 6 reps at 70% max weight
Set 4: 6 reps at 80% max weight

Tier 1: Deadlift
Barbell RDL - 3 sets of 10 reps

Tier 2: Lunge
Dumbbell Reverse Lunge - 3 sets of 10 reps per leg

Tier 3: Glute Bridge
Single Leg Glute Bridge - 3 sets of 10 reps per leg

WEEK 2
Workout #2: Upper Body/Bench Day

WORKOUT NOTES

- Circuit the mobility and core stability warm-up and limit to 10 minutes.

VARSITY LEVEL   OFF-SEASON I (SUMMER)

Target Area: Mobility/Core Stability Warm-Up
Dumbbell "T" Raise - 3 sets of 15 reps
Physioball Dead Bug - 3 sets of 8 super slow reps
PVC Bench Thoracic Extension - 3 sets for 30–45 seconds
Side Plank - 3 sets of 45 seconds per side

Tier 2: Throw
Medicine Ball Squat Press Throw - 3 sets of 5 reps

"Big 5" Strength
Dumbbell Bench Press (Eccentric)
Perform each rep with 4 seconds eccentric (slow and controlled movement
    down).
Set 1: 6 reps at 50% max weight
Set 2: 6 reps at 60% max weight
Set 3: 6 reps at 70% max weight
Set 4: 6 reps at 80% max weight

Upper Body Assistance
Barbell Row - 3 sets of 10 reps
Dumbbell Incline Chest Press - 3 sets of 10 reps

Tier 1: Body Weight Strength
TRX or Ring Row - 2 sets of 15 reps
Dumbbell Rear Delt Raise - 2 sets of 15 reps

Tier 2: Carry
Dumbbell or Trap Bar Farmer Walks - 3 sets of 40 yards

WEEK 2
Workout #3: Lower Body/Deadlift Day

WORKOUT NOTES

- Circuit the mobility and core stability warm-up and limit to 10 minutes.
- Consider adding weight to the barbell back box squat this week

Target Area: Mobility/Core Stability Warm-Up
Walking Lunge with Rotation - 3 sets of 12 reps per leg
Physioball Front Plank Circles - 3 sets for 30–45 seconds
Medicine Ball Thoracic Extension - 3 sets of 6 deep breaths
Alternate Leg Raise - 3 sets of 10 reps per leg

Tier 2: Lateral Jump (Isometric)
Lateral Squat Jump Isometric (stick and hold each landing for 2 seconds) - 3 sets
of 3 jumps in each direction

"Big 5" Strength
Trap Bar Deadlift (Eccentric)
Perform each rep with 4 seconds eccentric (slow and controlled movement
down).
Set 1: 6 reps at 50% max weight
Set 2: 6 reps at 60% max weight
Set 3: 6 reps at 70% max weight
Set 4: 6 reps at 80% max weight

Tier 1: Squat
Barbell Back Box Squat - 3 sets of 10 reps

Tier 2: Lunge
Dumbbell Lateral Lunge - 3 sets of 10 reps per leg

Tier 3: Leg Curl
Physioball Leg Curl - 2 sets of 12 reps

VARSITY LEVEL   OFF-SEASON I (SUMMER)

WEEK 2
Workout #4: Upper Body/Pull-Up Day

WORKOUT NOTES

- Circuit the mobility and core stability warm-up and limit to 10 minutes.
- If you cannot perform a full pull-up or chin-up, please substitute your pull-up/chin-up progression exercise into the "Big 5" strength section.
- Do as few sets as possible to accumulate the total pull-up/chin-up reps of the week, max 10 reps per set. Add a weight vest or chain after the athlete has progressed past 3 sets of 10 reps of body weight reps. Progress by either finishing 25 reps in fewer sets than last week OR by getting 30 pull-ups this week.

Target Area: Mobility/Core Stability Warm-Up
Dumbbell "T" Raise - 3 sets of 15 reps
Physioball Dead Bug - 3 sets of 8 super slow reps
PVC Bench Thoracic Extension - 3 sets for 30–45 seconds
Side Plank - 3 sets of 45 seconds per side

Tier 2: Rotation
Cable Chop or Medicine Ball Rotational Throw - 3 sets of 8 reps

"Big 5" Strength
Pull-Up/Chin-Up (weights optional) - 25 reps in as few sets as possible (see Workout Notes above)

Upper Body Assistance
Dumbbell Shoulder Press - 3 sets of 10 reps
One-Arm Dumbbell Row - 3 sets of 10 reps per arm

Tier 1: Body Weight Strength
TRX or Ring Push-Up - 2 sets of 12 reps
Dumbbell Lateral Raise - 2 sets of 15 reps

Tier 2: Carry
Dumbbell or Trap Bar Farmer Walks - 3 sets of 40 yards

WEEK 3
Workout #1: Lower Body/Squat Day

WORKOUT NOTES

- Circuit the mobility and core stability warm-up and limit to 10 minutes.
- Added volume (reps) to the assistance exercises

Target Area: Mobility/Core Stability Warm-Up
Walking Lunge with Rotation - 3 sets of 12 reps per leg
Physioball Front Plank Circles - 3 sets for 30–45 seconds
Medicine Ball Thoracic Extension - 3 sets of 6 deep breaths
Alternate Leg Raise - 3 sets of 10 reps per leg

Tier 2: Vertical Jump (Isometric)
Squat Jump Isometric (stick and hold each landing for 2 seconds) - 3 sets of 5
     jumps

"Big 5" Strength
Barbell Front Box Squat (Eccentric)
Perform each rep with 5 seconds eccentric (slow and controlled movement
     down).
Set 1: 3 reps at 45% max weight
Set 2: 3 reps at 55% max weight
Set 3: 3 reps at 65% max weight
Set 4: 3 reps at 75% max weight
Set 5: 3 reps at 85% max weight

Tier 1: Deadlift
Barbell RDL - 3 sets of 10 reps

Tier 2: Lunge
Dumbbell Reverse Lunge - 3 sets of 12 reps per leg

Tier 3: Glute Bridge
Single Leg Glute Bridge - 3 sets of 15 reps per leg

WEEK 3
Workout #2: Upper Body/Bench Day

WORKOUT NOTES
- Circuit the mobility and core stability warm-up and limit to 10 minutes.
- Added volume (reps) to the assistance exercises

Target Area: Mobility/Core Stability Warm-Up
Dumbbell "T" Raise - 3 sets of 15 reps
Physioball Dead Bug - 3 sets of 8 super slow reps
PVC Bench Thoracic Extension - 3 sets for 30–45 seconds
Side Plank - 3 sets of 45 seconds per side

Tier 2: Throw
Medicine Ball Squat Press Throw - 3 sets of 5 reps

"Big 5" Strength
Dumbbell Bench Press (Eccentric)
Perform each rep with 5 seconds eccentric (slow and controlled movement down).
Set 1: 3 reps at 45% max weight
Set 2: 3 reps at 55% max weight
Set 3: 3 reps at 65% max weight
Set 4: 3 reps at 75% max weight
Set 5: 3 reps at 85% max weight

Upper Body Assistance
Barbell Row - 3 sets of 10 reps
Dumbbell Incline Chest Press - 3 sets of 10 reps

Tier 1: Body Weight Strength
TRX or Ring Row - 2 sets of 20 reps
Dumbbell Rear Delt Raise - 2 sets of 20 reps

Tier 2: Carry
Dumbbell or Trap Bar Farmer Walks - 3 sets of 40 yards

WEEK 3
Workout #3: Lower Body/Deadlift Day

WORKOUT NOTES

- Circuit the mobility and core stability warm-up and limit to 10 minutes.
- Added volume (reps) to the assistance exercises

Target Area: Mobility/Core Stability Warm-Up
Walking Lunge with Rotation - 3 sets of 12 reps per leg
Physioball Front Plank Circles - 3 sets for 30–45 seconds
Medicine Ball Thoracic Extension - 3 sets of 6 deep breaths
Alternate Leg Raise - 3 sets of 10 reps per leg

Tier 2: Lateral Jump (Isometric)
Lateral Squat Jump Isometric (stick and hold each landing for 2 seconds) - 3 sets
of 3 jumps in each direction

"Big 5" Strength
Trap Bar Deadlift (Eccentric)
Perform each rep with 5 seconds eccentric (slow and controlled movement
down).
Set 1: 3 reps at 45% max weight
Set 2: 3 reps at 55% max weight
Set 3: 3 reps at 65% max weight
Set 4: 3 reps at 75% max weight
Set 5: 3 reps at 85% max weight

Tier 1: Squat
Barbell Back Box Squat - 3 sets of 10 reps

Tier 2: Lunge
Dumbbell Lateral Lunge - 3 sets of 10 reps per leg

Tier 3: Leg Curl
Physioball Leg Curl - 2 sets of 15 reps

WEEK 3
Workout #4: Upper Body/Pull-Up Day

WORKOUT NOTES

- Circuit the mobility and core stability warm-up and limit to 10 minutes.
- If you cannot perform a full pull-up or chin-up, please substitute your pull-up/chin-up progression exercise into the "Big 5" strength section.
- Do as few sets as possible to accumulate the total pull-up/chin-up reps of the week, max 10 reps per set. Add a weight vest or chain after the athlete has progressed past 3 sets of 10 reps of body weight reps. Progress by either finishing 25 reps in fewer sets than last week OR by getting 30 pull-ups this week.
- Added volume (reps) to the assistance exercises

Target Area: Mobility/Core Stability Warm-Up
Dumbbell "T" Raise - 3 sets of 15 reps
Physioball Dead Bug - 3 sets of 8 super slow reps
PVC Bench Thoracic Extension - 3 sets for 30–45 seconds
Side Plank - 3 sets of 45 seconds per side

Tier 2: Rotation
Cable Chop or Medicine Ball Rotational Throw - 3 sets of 8 reps

"Big 5" Strength
Pull-Up/Chin-Up (weights optional) - 25–30 reps in as few sets as possible (see Workout Notes above)

Upper Body Assistance
Dumbbell Shoulder Press - 3 sets of 10 reps
One-Arm Dumbbell Row - 3 sets of 10 reps per arm

Tier 1: Body Weight Strength
TRX or Ring Push-Up - 2 sets of 15 reps
Dumbbell Lateral Raise - 2 sets of 20 reps

Tier 2: Carry
Dumbbell or Trap Bar Farmer Walks - 3 sets of 40 yards

OFF-SEASON I [SUMMER]

VARSITY LEVEL

WEEK 4
Workout #1: Download Week

WORKOUT NOTES

- Volume (reps and sets) is cut in half
- Use only enough weight to teach the new movements
- Keep the rep speed slow and allow extra time to learn the new movements

Target Area: Mobility/Core Stability Warm-Up
Band Overhead Squat Pattern - 2 sets of 6 reps
Lunge Yoga Rotations - 1 set of 5 reps per side
Hang Knee or Leg Raise - 1 set of 6 reps

Tier 1: Strength
Barbell Back Box Squat (Eccentric) - 2 sets of 3 reps (3 seconds eccentric each rep)
Barbell Row (under hand grip) - 2 sets of 6 reps
Lateral Sled Walks - 1 set of 20 yards (2 each direction)
Dumbbell Rear Delt Raise - 1 set of 15 reps

Foam Roll Massage
10 minutes foam roll massage

WEEK 4
Workout #2: Download Week

WORKOUT NOTES

- Volume (reps and sets) is cut in half
- Use only enough weight to teach the new movements
- Keep the rep speed slow and allow extra time to learn the new movements

Target Area: Mobility/Core Stability Warm-Up
Yoga Push-Ups - 2 sets of 5 reps
Banded Dead Bug - 1 set of 8 reps per side (slow)
Side Plank with Leg Raise - 1 set of 6 reps per side

Tier 1: Strength
One-Arm Dumbbell Row or Landmine Row - 2 sets of 5 reps per arm
TRX Atomic Push-Up - 1 set of 8 reps
Dumbbell Single Leg RDL - 1 set of 5 reps per leg
Slider Leg Curl or Glute Ham Raise - 1 set of 8 reps

Foam Roll Massage
10 minutes foam roll massage

WEEK 4
Workout #3: Download Week

WORKOUT NOTES

- Volume (reps and sets) is cut in half
- Use only enough weight to teach the new movements
- Keep the rep speed slow and allow extra time to learn the new movements

Target Area: Mobility/Core Stability Warm-Up
PVC or Barbell Overhead Squat - 2 set of 5 reps
TRX or Ring Plank Fallouts - 2 sets of 6 reps

Tier 1: Strength
Barbell Glute Bridge or Barbell Hip Thrust - 1 set of 10 reps
Barbell Sumo Deadlift - 2 sets of 3 reps
Spiderman Push-Up - 1 set of 12 reps
Single Arm Front Rack Farmer Walk - 1 set of 40 yards per side

Foam Roll Massage
10 minutes foam roll massage

WEEK 5
Workout #1: Lower Body/Squat Day

WORKOUT NOTES

- Circuit the mobility and core stability warm-up and limit to 10 minutes.
- Elevate the sumo deadlift (blocks or rack) off the floor if necessary.

Target Area: Mobility/Core Stability Warm-Up
Band Overhead Squat Pattern - 3 sets of 12 reps
TRX or Ring Plank Fallouts - 3 sets of 12 reps
Lunge Yoga Rotations - 3 sets of 8 reps per side
Hang Knee or Leg Raise - 3 sets of 12 reps

Tier 2: Lateral Jump (Isometric)
Broad Jump Isometric (hold each landing for 3 seconds) - 3 sets of 5 reps

"Big 5" Strength
Barbell Back Box Squat (Eccentric)
Perform each rep with 3 seconds eccentric (slow and controlled movement
     down).
Set 1: 8 reps at 45% max weight
Set 2: 8 reps at 55% max weight
Set 3: 8 reps at 65% max weight
Set 4: 8 reps at 75% max weight

Tier 1: Deadlift
Barbell Sumo Deadlift - 3 sets of 6 reps

Tier 2: Lunge
Dumbbell Single Leg RDL - 3 sets of 10 reps per leg

Tier 3: Leg Curl
Slider Leg Curl or Glute Ham Raise - 2 sets of 10 reps

OFF-SEASON I (SUMMER)   VARSITY LEVEL

WEEK 5
Workout #2: Upper Body/Shoulder Press Day

WORKOUT NOTES

- Circuit the mobility and core stability warm-up and limit to 10 minutes.

Target Area: Mobility/Core Stability Warm-Up
Yoga Push-Ups - 3 sets of 15 reps
Banded Dead Bug - 3 sets of 8 super slow reps per side
PVC or Barbell Overhead Squat - 3 sets of 10 reps
Side Plank with Leg Raise - 3 sets of 12 reps per side

Tier 2: Rotation
Cable Lift or Medicine Ball Lateral Bound to Rotational Throw - 3 sets of 8 reps
     per side

"Big 5" Strength
Dumbbell Shoulder Press (Eccentric)
Perform each rep with 3 seconds eccentric (slow and controlled movement
     down).
Set 1: 8 reps at 45% max weight
Set 2: 8 reps at 55% max weight
Set 3: 8 reps at 65% max weight
Set 4: 8 reps at 75% max weight

Upper Body Assistance
One-Arm Dumbbell Row or Landmine Row - 3 sets of 10 reps per arm
Cable Face Pull - 3 sets of 15 reps

Tier 1: Body Weight Strength
Spiderman Push-Up - 2 sets of 12 reps
Dumbbell Rear Delt Raise - 2 sets of 15 reps

Tier 2: Carry
Single Arm Front Rack Farmer Walk - 3 sets of 40 yards per side

WEEK 5
Workout #3: Lower Body/Deadlift Day

WORKOUT NOTES

- Circuit the mobility and core stability warm-up and limit to 10 minutes.
- Set up rack or block height in order to maintain a neutral/slight arch in the lower back for the deadlift. For most, that is 4–8 inches off the floor.

Target Area: Mobility/Core Stability Warm-Up
Band Overhead Squat Pattern - 3 sets of 12 reps
TRX or Ring Plank Fallouts - 3 sets of 12 reps
Lunge Yoga Rotations - 3 sets of 8 reps per side
Hang Knee or Leg Raise - 3 sets of 12 reps

Tier 2: Lateral Jump (Isometric)
Single Leg Lateral Jump to a Double Leg Landing Isometric - 3 sets of 3 jumps
    per side

"Big 5" Strength
Barbell Rack or Block Deadlift (Eccentric)
Perform each rep with 3 seconds eccentric (slow and controlled movement
    down).
Set 1: 8 reps at 45% max weight
Set 2: 8 reps at 55% max weight
Set 3: 8 reps at 65% max weight
Set 4: 8 reps at 75% max weight

Tier 1: Squat
Dumbbell Goblet Pause Squat - 3 sets of 5 reps (3 second pause per rep)

Tier 2: Lunge
Lateral Sled Walks - 4 sets of 20 yards (2 reps per direction)

Tier 3: Glute Bridge
Barbell Glute Bridge or Barbell Hip Thrust - 3 sets of 10 reps

OFF-SEASON I (SUMMER)

VARSITY LEVEL

WEEK 5
Workout #4: Upper Body/Pull-Up Day

WORKOUT NOTES

- Circuit the mobility and core stability warm-up and limit to 10 minutes.
- If the athlete cannot perform a full pull-up or chin-up, please substitute their pull-up/chin-up progression exercise into the "Big 5" strength section.
- Do as few sets as possible to accumulate the total pull-up/chin-up reps of the week, max 10 reps per set. Add a weight vest or chain after the athlete has progressed past 3 sets of 10 reps of body weight reps.

Target Area: Mobility/Core Stability Warm-Up
Yoga Push-Ups - 3 sets of 15 reps
Banded Dead Bug - 3 sets of 8 super slow reps per side
PVC or Barbell Overhead Squat - 3 sets of 10 reps
Side Plank + Leg Raise - 3 sets of 12 reps per side

Tier 2: Throw
Medicine Ball Reverse Scoop Throw for distance - 3 sets of 5 reps

"Big 5" Strength
Pull-Up/Chin-Up (weights optional) - 30 reps in as few sets as possible (see
    Workout Notes above)

Upper Body Assistance
Dumbbell Single Arm Bench Press - 3 sets of 10 reps per arm
Barbell Row (under hand grip) - 3 sets of 10 reps

Tier 1: Body Weight Strength
TRX Atomic Push-Up - 2 sets of 12 reps
Dumbbell Lateral Raise - 2 sets of 15 reps

Tier 2: Carry
Single Arm Front Rack Farmer Walk - 3 sets of 40 yards per side

WEEK 6
Workout #1: Lower Body/Squat Day

WORKOUT NOTES

- Circuit the mobility and core stability warm-up and limit to 10 minutes.
- Lower the sumo deadlift (blocks or rack) to the floor before adding weight.

Target Area: Mobility/Core Stability Warm-Up
Band Overhead Squat Pattern - 3 sets of 12 reps
TRX or Ring Plank Fallouts - 3 sets of 12 reps
Lunge Yoga Rotations - 3 sets of 8 reps per side
Hang Knee or Leg Raise - 3 sets of 12 reps

Tier 2: Lateral Jump (Isometric)
Broad Jump Isometric (hold each landing for 3 seconds) - 3 sets of 5 reps

"Big 5" Strength
Barbell Back Box Squat (Eccentric)
Perform each rep with 4 seconds eccentric (slow and controlled movement
    down).
Set 1: 6 reps at 50% max weight
Set 2: 6 reps at 60% max weight
Set 3: 6 reps at 70% max weight
Set 4: 6 reps at 80% max weight

Tier 1: Deadlift
Barbell Sumo Deadlift - 3 sets of 6 reps

Tier 2: Lunge
Dumbbell Single Leg RDL - 3 sets of 10 reps per leg

Tier 3: Leg Curl
Slider Leg Curl or Glute Ham Raise - 2 sets of 10 reps

WEEK 6
Workout #2: Upper Body/Shoulder Press Day

WORKOUT NOTES

- Circuit the mobility and core stability warm-up and limit to 10 minutes.

Target Area: Mobility/Core Stability Warm-Up
Yoga Push-Ups - 3 sets of 15 reps
Banded Dead Bug - 3 sets of 8 super slow reps per side
PVC or Barbell Overhead Squat - 3 sets of 10 reps
Side Plank with Leg Raise - 3 sets of 12 reps per side

Tier 2: Rotation
Cable Lift or Medicine Ball Lateral Bound to Rotational Throw - 3 sets of 8 reps
    per side

"Big 5" Strength
Dumbbell Shoulder Press (Eccentric)
Perform each rep with 4 seconds eccentric (slow and controlled movement
    down).
Set 1: 6 reps at 50% max weight
Set 2: 6 reps at 60% max weight
Set 3: 6 reps at 70% max weight
Set 4: 6 reps at 80% max weight

Upper Body Assistance
One-Arm Dumbbell Row or Landmine Row - 3 sets of 10 reps per arm
Cable Face Pull - 3 sets of 15 reps

Tier 1: Body Weight Strength
Spiderman Push-Up - 2 sets of 12 reps
Dumbbell Rear Delt Raise - 2 sets of 15 reps

Tier 2: Carry
Single Arm Front Rack Farmer Walk - 3 sets of 40 yards per side

WEEK 6
Workout #3: Lower Body/Deadlift Day

WORKOUT NOTES

- Circuit the mobility and core stability warm-up and limit to 10 minutes.
- Set up rack or block height in order to maintain a neutral/slight arch in the lower back for the deadlift. For most, that is 4–8 inches off the floor.

OFF-SEASON I (SUMMER)

VARSITY LEVEL

Target Area: Mobility/Core Stability Warm-Up
Band Overhead Squat Pattern - 3 sets of 12 reps
TRX or Ring Plank Fallouts - 3 sets of 12 reps
Lunge Yoga Rotations - 3 sets of 8 reps per side
Hang Knee or Leg Raise - 3 of 12 reps

Tier 2: Lateral Jump (Isometric)
Single Leg Lateral Jump to a Double Leg Landing Isometric - 3 sets of 3 jumps
per side

"Big 5" Strength
Barbell Rack or Block Deadlift (Eccentric)
Perform each rep with 4 seconds eccentric (slow and controlled movement
down).
Set 1: 6 reps at 50% max weight
Set 2: 6 reps at 60% max weight
Set 3: 6 reps at 70% max weight
Set 4: 6 reps at 80% max weight

Tier 1: Squat
Dumbbell Goblet Pause Squat - 3 sets of 5 reps (3 second pause per rep)

Tier 2: Lunge
Lateral Sled Walks - 4 sets of 20 yards (2 in each direction)

Tier 3: Glute Bridge
Barbell Glute Bridge or Barbell Hip Thrust - 3 sets of 10 reps

WEEK 6
Workout #4: Upper Body/Pull-Up Day

WORKOUT NOTES

- Circuit the mobility and core stability warm-up and limit to 10 minutes.
- If you cannot perform a full pull-up or chin-up, please substitute your pull-up/chin-up progression exercise into the "Big 5" strength section.
- Do as few sets as possible to accumulate the total pull-up/chin-up reps of the week, max 10 reps per set. Add a weight vest or chain after the athlete has progressed past 3 sets of 10 reps of body weight reps. Progress by either finishing 25 reps in fewer sets than last week OR by getting 30 pull-ups this week.

Target Area: Mobility/Core Stability Warm-Up
Yoga Push-Ups - 3 sets of 15 reps
Banded Dead Bug - 3 sets of 8 super slow reps per side
PVC or Barbell Overhead Squat - 3 sets of 10 reps
Side Plank with Leg Raise - 3 sets of 12 reps per side

Tier 2: Throw
Medicine Ball Reverse Scoop Throw (for distance) - 3 sets of 5 reps

"Big 5" Strength
Pull-Up/Chin-Up (weights optional) - 30 reps in as few sets as possible (see Workout Notes above)

Upper Body Assistance
Dumbbell Single Arm Bench Press - 3 sets of 10 reps per arm
Barbell Row (under hand grip) - 3 sets of 10 reps

Tier 1: Body Weight Strength
TRX Atomic Push-Up - 2 sets of 12 reps
Dumbbell Lateral Raise - 2 sets of 15 reps

Tier 2: Carry
Single Arm Front Rack Farmer Walk - 3 sets of 40 yards per side

WEEK 7
Workout #1: Lower Body/Squat Day

WORKOUT NOTES

- Circuit the mobility and core stability warm-up and limit to 10 minutes.
- Lower the sumo deadlift (blocks or rack) to the floor before adding weight.
- Added volume to the assistance work

Target Area: Mobility/Core Stability Warm-Up
Band Overhead Squat Pattern - 3 sets of 12 reps
TRX or Ring Plank Fallouts - 3 sets of 12 reps
Lunge Yoga Rotations - 3 sets of 8 reps per side
Hang Knee or Leg Raise - 3 sets of 12 reps

Tier 2: Lateral Jump (Isometric)
Broad Jump Isometric (hold each landing for 3 seconds) - 3 sets of 5 reps

"Big 5" Strength
Barbell Back Box Squat (Eccentric)
Perform each rep with 5 seconds eccentric (slow and controlled movement down).
Set 1: 3 reps at 45% max weight
Set 2: 3 reps at 55% max weight
Set 3: 3 reps at 65% max weight
Set 4: 3 reps at 75% max weight
Set 5: 3 reps at 85% max weight

Tier 1: Deadlift
Barbell Sumo Deadlift - 3 sets of 6 reps

Tier 2: Lunge
Dumbbell Single Leg RDL - 4 sets of 8 reps per leg

Tier 3: Leg Curl
Slider Leg Curl or Glute Ham Raise - 3 sets of 10 reps

WEEK 7
Workout #2: Upper Body/Shoulder Press Day

WORKOUT NOTES

- Circuit the mobility and core stability warm-up and limit to 10 minutes.
- Added volume to the assistance work

Target Area: Mobility/Core Stability Warm-Up
Yoga Push-Ups - 3 sets of 15 reps
Banded Dead Bug - 3 sets of 8 super slow reps per side
PVC or Barbell Overhead Squat - 3 sets of 10 reps
Side Plank with Leg Raise - 3 sets of 12 reps per side

Tier 2: Rotation
Cable Lift or Medicine Ball Lateral Bound to Rotational Throw - 3 sets of 8 reps
per side

"Big 5" Strength
Dumbbell Shoulder Press (Eccentric)
Perform each rep with 5 seconds eccentric (slow and controlled movement
down).
Set 1: 3 reps at 45% max weight
Set 2: 3 reps at 55% max weight
Set 3: 3 reps at 65% max weight
Set 4: 3 reps at 75% max weight
Set 5: 3 reps at 85% max weight

Upper Body Assistance
One-Arm Dumbbell Row or Landmine Row - 3 sets of 10 reps per arm
Cable Face Pull - 3 sets of 15 reps

Tier 1: Body Weight Strength
Spiderman Push-Up - 3 sets of 12 reps
Dumbbell Rear Delt Raise - 3 sets of 15 reps

Tier 2: Carry
Single Arm Front Rack Farmer Walk - 3 sets of 40 yards per side

WEEK 7
Workout #3: Lower Body/Deadlift Day

WORKOUT NOTES

- Circuit the mobility and core stability warm-up and limit to 10 minutes.
- Set up rack or block height in order to maintain a neutral/slight arch in the lower back for the deadlift. For most people, that is 4–8 inches off the floor.
- Added volume to the assistance work

OFF-SEASON I (SUMMER)

VARSITY LEVEL

Target Area: Mobility/Core Stability Warm-Up
Band Overhead Squat Pattern - 3 sets of 12 reps
TRX or Ring Plank Fallouts - 3 sets of 12 reps
Lunge Yoga Rotations - 3 sets of 8 reps per side
Hang Knee or Leg Raise - 3 sets of 12 reps

Tier 2: Lateral Jump (Isometric)
Single Leg Lateral Jump to a Double Leg Landing Isometric - 3 sets of 3 jumps per side

"Big 5" Strength
Barbell Rack or Block Deadlift (Eccentric)
Perform each rep with 5 seconds eccentric (slow and controlled movement down).
Set 1: 3 reps at 45% max weight
Set 2: 3 reps at 55% max weight
Set 3: 3 reps at 65% max weight
Set 4: 3 reps at 75% max weight
Set 5: 3 reps at 85% max weight

Tier 1: Squat
Dumbbell Goblet Pause Squat - 4 sets of 5 reps (3 second pause per rep)

Tier 2: Lunge
Lateral Sled Walks - 6 sets of 20 yards (3 reps per direction)

Tier 3: Glute Bridge
Barbell Glute Bridge or Barbell Hip Thrust - 3 sets of 10 reps

WEEK 7
Workout #4: Upper Body/Pull-Up Day

WORKOUT NOTES

- Circuit the mobility and core stability warm-up and limit to 10 minutes.
- If the athlete cannot perform a full pull-up or chin-up, please substitute their pull-up/chin-up progression exercise into the "Big 5" strength section.
- Do as few sets as possible to accumulate the total pull-up/chin-up reps of the week, max 10 reps per set. Add a weight vest or chain after the athlete has progressed past 3 sets of 10 reps of body weight reps. Progress by either finishing 25 reps in fewer sets than last week OR by getting 30 pull-ups this week.
- Added volume to the assistance work

Target Area: Mobility/Core Stability Warm-Up
Yoga Push-Ups - 3 sets of 15 reps
Banded Dead Bug - 3 sets of 8 super slow reps per side
PVC or Barbell Overhead Squat - 3 sets of 10 reps
Side Plank with Leg Raise - 3 sets of 12 reps per side

Tier 2: Throw
Medicine Ball Reverse Scoop Throw for distance - 3 sets of 5 reps

"Big 5" Strength
Pull-Up/Chin-Up (weights optional) - 30 reps in as few sets as possible (see Workout Notes above)

Upper Body Assistance
Dumbbell Single Arm Bench Press - 3 sets of 10 reps per arm
Barbell Row (under hand grip) - 3 sets of 10 reps

Tier 1: Body Weight Strength
TRX Atomic Push-Up - 3 sets of 12 reps
Dumbbell Lateral Raise - 3 sets of 15 reps

Tier 2: Carry
Single Arm Front Rack Farmer Walk - 3 sets of 40 yards per side

OFF-SEASON II (FALL)

N ow we transition to the second phase of off-season programming, as players return to school for the fall season. Many strength and conditioning coaches consider these to be the most impactful months of training, and place a greater emphasis on power while conditioning work is made optional based on travel baseball schedules.

In this section, we make use of PAP power sets and dynamic effort sets to build explosive power. **Post activation potentiation (PAP) sets** are a go-to method for many high-level athletes which pair a heavy compound exercise (a dumbbell chest press, for example) with a lighter, dynamic exercise (such as plyometric push-ups). By combining a strength exercise at 75–85 percent of max with a similar power exercise, you build explosive power. Dynamic effort (DE) sets, on the other hand, build strength and speed by working at a moderate intensity (55–70 percent) with max bar speed for only 2–3 reps for 8–10 sets.

Over the next 8 weeks, we rotate the exercises used for PAP power and dynamic effort while introducing new speed drills. We also begin using **repetition effort (RE)** techniques for "Fun" Fridays! Repetition effort builds massive size by working at a moderate intensity (65–75 percent) for only higher volumes of 8–12 reps for 3–5 sets. Finally, we introduce Medicine Ball Tennis for healthy competition, functional core rotation strength, and conditioning.

Program Breakdown

Monday	Wednesday	Friday
Target Area: Activation/ Mobility Warm-Up	**Target Area:** Activation/ Mobility Warm-Up	**Target Area:** Activation/ Mobility Warm-Up
Target Area: Acceleration	**Target Area:** Reaction Agility	**Target Area:** Sprint
Target Area: Reaction Agility	**Target Area:** Sprint	**Target Area:** Change of Direction
Intensity Technique: Dynamic Effort Push Press	**Intensity Technique:** PAP Power Pull-Up/Chin-Up	**"Big 5" Strength** Bench
Intensity Technique: PAP Power Front Squat	**Intensity Technique:** Dynamic Effort Trap Bar Deadlift	**Tier 2:** Assistance Lower Body Pull Upper Body Pull
Tier 2: Assistance Lower Body Pull Upper Body Pull	**Tier 2:** Assistance Lower Body Pull Upper Body Push	**Upper Body** Fun Friday and Medicine Ball Tennis

PROGRAM NOTES

- This phase is programmed for three workouts a week and does not include a download week to accommodate for most fall ball schedules and the addition of academic work now that school has started. A typical fall ball schedule will most likely create natural periods of recovery due to missed workouts, while the addition of academic work makes three workouts a week perfect.

- However, the first week of this program is still intended to help ease the transition into fall workouts from the end of the summer.

- Speed development (acceleration, reaction agility, sprint, and change of direction) is programmed first to place an emphasis on power and speed.

- "Fun" Fridays include conditioning games (Medicine Ball Tennis) and competitions, giving the players something to look forward to in order to help keep energy and morale levels high. (See page 319 for the rules to Medicine Ball Tennis.)

WEEK 1
Workout #1: Transition Week

WORKOUT NOTES

- Lower volume and intensity for the first week back
- The 4-Way Pull-Up listed in the upper body segment refers to performing a 1) Wide Grip Pull-Up, 2) Traditional Pull-Up, 3) Neutral Grip Pull-Up and 4) Chin-Up, in that sequence, as a mechanical drop set. Perform for equal number of reps per exercise, starting with 1 rep.

Target Area: Activation/Mobility Warm-Up
PVC or Barbell Overhead Squat - 3 sets of 5 reps with 3 second pause
Dumbbell "T" Raise (Rear Delt Raise) - 3 sets of 12 reps

Target Area: Acceleration
Moderate Sled Push (30-50% of body weight) - 6 sets of 20 yards

Intensity Technique: Dynamic Effort
Dumbbell Single Arm Push Press - 3 sets of 3 reps each arm at 60% max weight

Intensity Technique: PAP Power
Alternate sets:
1A. Barbell Front Squat - 3 sets of 3 reps at 70% max weight
1B. Squat Jump - 3 sets of 5 reps

Tier 2: Assistance
Glute Ham Raise - 2 sets of 12 reps
4-Way Pull-Up (see Workout Notes) - 2 or 3 sets

VARSITY LEVEL   OFF-SEASON II (FALL)

WEEK 1
Workout #2: Transition Week

WORKOUT NOTES

- Lower volume and intensity for the first week back

Target Area: Activation/Mobility Warm-Up
Lunge Yoga Rotations - 3 sets of 12 reps each
Foam Roll Latissimus Dorsi (Lat) Muscles - 3 sets of 30 seconds per side

Intensity Technique: PAP Power
Alternate sets:
1A. Pull-Up/Chin-Up - 3 sets of 5 reps
1B. Medicine Ball Overhead Throw - 3 sets of 5 reps

Intensity Technique: Dynamic Effort
Trap Bar Deadlift - 3 sets of 3 reps at 60% max weight

Tier 2: Assistance
Slider Single Leg Curl - 2 sets of 8 reps per leg
Lunge Dumbbell Shoulder Press - 2 sets of 8 reps

OFF-SEASON II (FALL)   VARSITY LEVEL

WEEK 1
Workout #3: Transition Week

WORKOUT NOTES

- Lower volume and intensity for the first week back
- For the Bicep Blaster Super Set (combination chin-up/dumbbell bicep curl), do 70% of your max chin-ups (leaving 2–3 reps in the tank). Immediately super set that with a dumbbell bicep curl. If you can do more than 12 reps of the bicep curls, either do more chin-ups or grab heavier dumbbells.

Target Area: Activation/Mobility Warm-Up
Band Pull-Aparts - 3 sets of 25 reps
Yoga Push-Up - 3 sets of 10 reps

"Big 5" Strength
Dumbbell Single Arm Bench Press
Set 1: 5 reps each arm at 45% max weight
Set 2: 5 reps each arm at 55% max weight
Set 3: 5 reps each arm at 65% max weight
Set 4: 5 reps each arm at 75% max weight

Tier 2: Assistance
Kettlebell Sumo Deadlift - 2 sets of 8 reps
Dumbbell Farmer Walk - 2 sets of 40 yards

Upper Body: "Fun" Friday
Bicep Blaster Super Set (Chin-Up/Dumbbell Bicep Hammer Curl) - 2–3 sets
Cable Rope Triceps Extensions - 2 sets of 12 reps

WEEK 2
Workout #1: Vertical Power

WORKOUT NOTES

- Additional speed development drills
- The 4-Way Pull-Up listed in the upper body segment refers to performing a 1) Wide Grip Pull-Up, 2) Traditional Pull-Up, 3) Neutral Grip Pull-Up and 4) Chin-Up, in that sequence, as a mechanical drop set. Perform for equal number of reps per exercise, starting with 1 rep.

Target Area: Activation/Mobility Warm-Up
PVC or Barbell Overhead Squat - 3 sets of 5 reps with 3 second pause
Dumbbell "T" Raise (Rear Delt Raise) - 3 sets of 12 reps

Target Area: Acceleration
Moderate Sled Push (30–50% of body weight) - 6 sets of 20 yards

Target Area: Reaction Agility (Visual)
Partner Mirror Lateral Movement Drill (within 5 yard cones) - 4 sets

Intensity Technique: Dynamic Effort
Dumbbell Single Arm Push Press - 3 sets of 3 reps each arm at 60% max weight

Intensity Technique: PAP Power
Alternate sets:
1A. Barbell Front Squat - 3 sets of 3 reps at 70% max weight
1B. Squat Jump - 3 sets of 5 reps

Tier 2: Assistance
Glute Ham Raise - 2 sets of 12 reps
4-Way Pull-Up – 2 or 3 sets

WEEK 2
Workout #2: Pull-Up and Deadlift Power

WORKOUT NOTES

- Additional speed development drills

Target Area: Activation/Mobility Warm-Up
Lunge Yoga Rotations - 3 sets of 12 reps each
Foam Roll Latissimus Dorsi (Lat) Muscles - 3 sets of 30 seconds each side

Target Area: Reaction Agility (Verbal)
3-cone drill on "WHISTLE" - 4 sets

Target Area: Sprint
Circle Chase Sprints - 3 sprints in each direction
One athlete starts 3–5 yards in front of another. The other chases. On "GO," the athlete has to slap/catch the athlete in front.

Intensity Technique: PAP Power
Alternate sets:
1A. Pull-Up/Chin-Up - 3 sets of 5 reps
1B. Medicine Ball Overhead Throw - 3 sets of 5 reps

Intensity Technique: Dynamic Effort
Trap Bar Deadlift - 3 sets of 3 reps at 60% max weight

Tier 2: Assistance
Slider Single Leg Curl - 2 sets of 8 reps per leg
Lunge Dumbbell Shoulder Press - 2 sets of 8 reps

WEEK 2
Workout #3: "Fun" Friday

WORKOUT NOTES

- Additional speed development drills
- For the Bicep Blaster Super Set (combination chin-up/dumbbell bicep curl), do 70% of your max chin-ups (leaving 2–3 reps in the tank). Immediately super set that with a dumbbell bicep curl. If you can do more than 12 reps of the bicep curls, either do more chin-ups or grab heavier dumbbells.

Target Area: Activation/Mobility Warm-Up
Band Pull-Aparts - 3 sets of 25 reps
Yoga Push-Up - 3 sets of 10 reps

Target Area: Sprint
20-yard Swim Noodle Chase Drill - 4 sets
One athlete starts 3–5 yards in front of another. The other chases, holding a swim noodle. On "GO," the athlete with the swim noodle has to slap/catch the athlete in front before he reaches 20 yards.

Target Area: Change of Direction
Ice Skater Jump to Forward Sprint - 4 total sprints

"Big 5" Strength
Dumbbell Single Arm Bench Press
Set 1: 5 reps each arm at 45% max weight
Set 2: 5 reps each arm at 55% max weight
Set 3: 5 reps each arm at 65% max weight
Set 4: 5 reps each arm at 75% max weight

Tier 2: Assistance
Kettlebell Sumo Deadlift - 2 sets of 8 reps
Dumbbell Farmer Walk - 2 sets of 40 yards

Upper Body: "Fun" Friday
Bicep Blaster Super Set (Chin-Up/Dumbbell Bicep Hammer Curl) - 2–3 sets
Cable Rope Triceps Extensions - 2 sets of 12 reps

Optional Conditioning Game
Medicine Ball Tennis

WEEK 3
Workout #1: Vertical Power

WORKOUT NOTES

- More volume (reps and sets) in the weight room
- The 4-Way Pull-Up listed in the upper body segment refers to performing a 1) Wide Grip Pull-Up, 2) Traditional Pull-Up, 3) Neutral Grip Pull-Up and 4) Chin-Up, in that sequence, as a mechanical drop set. Perform for equal number of reps per exercise, starting with 1 rep.

Target Area: Activation/Mobility Warm-Up
PVC or Barbell Overhead Squat - 3 sets of 5 reps with 3 second pause
Dumbbell "T" Raise (Rear Delt Raise) - 3 sets of 12 reps

Target Area: Acceleration
Moderate Sled Push (30–50% of body weight) - 6 sets of 20 yards

Target Area: Reaction Agility (Visual)
Partner Mirror Lateral Movement Drill (within 5 yard cones) - 4 sets

Intensity Technique: Dynamic Effort
Dumbbell Single Arm Push Press - 4 sets of 3 reps each arm at 60% max weight

Intensity Technique: PAP Power
Alternate sets:
1A. Barbell Front Squat - 3 sets of 5 reps at 70% max weight
1B. Squat Jump - 3 sets of 5 reps

Tier 2: Assistance
Glute Ham Raise - 3 sets of 12 reps
4-Way Pull-Up - 2 or 3 sets

OFF-SEASON II (FALL)

VARSITY LEVEL

WEEK 3
Workout #2: Pull-Up and Deadlift Power

WORKOUT NOTES

- More volume (reps and sets) in the weight room

Target Area: Activation/Mobility Warm-Up
Lunge Yoga Rotations - 3 sets of 12 reps each
Foam Roll Latissimus Dorsi (Lat) Muscles - 3 sets of 30 seconds per side

Target Area: Reaction Agility (Verbal)
3-cone drill on "WHISTLE" - 4 sets

Target Area: Sprint
Circle Chase Sprints - 3 sprints in each direction
One athlete starts 3–5 yards in front of another. The other chases. On "GO," the
    athlete has to slap/catch the athlete in front.

Intensity Technique: PAP Power
Alternate sets:
1A. Pull-Up/Chin-Up - 3 sets of 8 reps
1B. Medicine Ball Overhead Throw - 3 sets of 5 reps

Intensity Technique: Dynamic Effort
Trap Bar Deadlift - 3 sets of 5 reps at 60% max weight

Tier 2: Assistance
Slider Single Leg Curl - 3 sets of 8 reps per leg
Lunge Dumbbell Shoulder Press - 3 sets of 8 reps

WEEK 3
Workout #3: "Fun" Friday

WORKOUT NOTES

- More volume (reps and sets) in the weight room
- For the Bicep Blaster Super Set (combination chin-up/dumbbell bicep curl), do 70% of your max chin-ups (leaving 2–3 reps in the tank). Immediately super set that with a dumbbell bicep curl. If you can do more than 12 reps of the bicep curls, either do more chin-ups or grab heavier dumbbells.

Target Area: Activation/Mobility Warm-Up
Band Pull-Aparts - 3 sets of 25 reps
Yoga Push-Up - 3 sets of 10 reps

Target Area: Sprint
20-yard Swim Noodle Chase Drill - 4 sets
One athlete starts 3–5 yards in front of another. The other chases, holding a swim noodle. On "GO," the athlete with the swim noodle has to slap/catch the athlete in front before he reaches 20 yards.

Target Area: Change of Direction
Ice Skater Jump to Forward Sprint - 4 total sprints

"Big 5" Strength
Dumbbell Single Arm Bench Press
Set 1: 5 reps each arm at 50% max weight
Set 2: 8 reps each arm at 75% max weight
Set 3: 8 reps each arm at 75% max weight
Set 4: 8 reps each arm at 75% max weight

Tier 2: Assistance
Kettlebell Sumo Deadlift - 2 sets of 8 reps
Dumbbell Farmer Walk - 2 sets of 40 yards

Upper Body: "Fun" Friday
Bicep Blaster Super Set (Chin-Up/Dumbbell Bicep Hammer Curl) - 2–3 sets
Cable Rope Triceps Extensions - 2 sets of 12 reps

Optional Conditioning Game
Medicine Ball Tennis

WEEK 4
Workout #1: Vertical Power

WORKOUT NOTES

- More volume (reps and sets) for the Speed Drills
- The 4-Way Pull-Up listed in the upper body segment refers to performing a 1) Wide Grip Pull-Up, 2) Traditional Pull-Up, 3) Neutral Grip Pull-Up and 4) Chin-Up, in that sequence, as a mechanical drop set. Perform for equal number of reps per exercise, starting with 1 rep.

Target Area: Activation/Mobility Warm-Up
PVC or Barbell Overhead Squat - 3 sets of 5 reps with 3 second pause
Dumbbell "T" Raise (Rear Delt Raise) - 3 sets of 12 reps

Target Area: Acceleration
Moderate Sled Push (30–50% of body weight) - 8 sets of 20 yards

Target Area: Reaction Agility (Visual)
Partner Mirror Lateral Movement Drill (within 5 yard cones) - 6 sets

Intensity Technique: Dynamic Effort
Dumbbell Single Arm Push Press - 4 sets of 3 reps each arm at 60% max weight

Intensity Technique: PAP Power
Alternate sets:
1A. Barbell Front Squat - 3 sets of 5 reps at 70% max weight
1B. Squat Jump - 3 sets of 5 reps

Tier 2: Assistance
Glute Ham Raise - 3 sets of 12 reps
4-Way Pull-Up - 3 sets of AMRAP

WEEK 4
Workout #2: Pull-Up and Deadlift Power

WORKOUT NOTES

- More volume (reps and sets) for the Speed Drills

Target Area: Activation/Mobility Warm-Up
Lunge Yoga Rotations - 3 sets of 12 reps each
Foam Roll Latissimus Dorsi (Lat) Muscles - 3 sets of 30 seconds per side

Target Area: Reaction Agility (Verbal)
3-cone drill on "WHISTLE" - 6 sets

Target Area: Sprint
Circle Chase Sprints - 4 sprints in each direction
One athlete starts 3–5 yards in front of another. The other chases. On "GO", the athlete has to slap/catch the athlete in front.

Intensity Technique: PAP Power
Alternate sets:
1A. Pull-Up/Chin-Up - 3 sets of 8 reps
1B. Medicine Ball Overhead Throw - 3 sets of 5 reps

Intensity Technique: Dynamic Effort
Trap Bar Deadlift - 3 sets of 5 reps at 60% max weight

Tier 2: Assistance
Slider Single Leg Curl - 3 sets of 8 reps per leg
Lunge Dumbbell Shoulder Press - 3 sets of 8 reps

WEEK 4
Workout #3: "Fun" Friday

WORKOUT NOTES

- More volume (reps and sets) for the Speed Drills
- For the Bicep Blaster Super Set (combination chin-up/dumbbell bicep curl), do 70% of your max chin-ups (leaving 2–3 reps in the tank). Immediately super set that with a dumbbell bicep curl. If you can do more than 12 reps of the bicep curls, either do more chin-ups or grab heavier dumbbells.

Target Area: Activation/Mobility Warm-Up
Band Pull-Aparts - 3 sets of 25 reps
Yoga Push-Up - 3 sets of 10 reps

Target Area: Sprint
20-yard Swim Noodle Chase Drill - 6 sets
One athlete starts 3–5 yards in front of another. The other chases, holding a swim noodle. On "GO," the athlete with the swim noodle has to slap/catch the athlete in front before he reaches 20 yards.

Target Area: Change of Direction
Ice Skater Jump to Forward Sprint - 6 total sprints

"Big 5" Strength
Dumbbell Single Arm Bench Press
Set 1: 5 reps each arm at 50% max weight
Set 2: 8 reps each arm at 75% max weight
Set 3: 8 reps each arm at 75% max weight
Set 4: 8 reps each arm at 75% max weight

Tier 2: Assistance
Kettlebell Sumo Deadlift - 2 sets of 8 reps
Dumbbell Farmer Walk - 2 sets of 40 yards

Upper Body: "Fun" Friday
Bicep Blaster Super Set (Chin-Up/Dumbbell Bicep Hammer Curl) - 2–3 sets
Cable Rope Triceps Extensions - 2 sets of 12 reps

Optional Conditioning Game
Medicine Ball Tennis

WEEK 5
Workout #1: Vertical Power

WORKOUT NOTES

- New variations of speed development drills, plyometric exercise in PAP set, new assistance exercise.

Target Area: Activation/Mobility Warm-Up
PVC or Barbell Overhead Squat - 3 sets of 5 reps with 3 second pause
Dumbbell "T" Raise (Rear Delt Raise) - 3 sets of 12 reps

Target Area: Acceleration
Sled Push Sprint (10–30% of body weight) - 6 sets of 20 yards

Target Area: Reaction Agility (Visual)
Partner 5-yard backpedal sprint to 5-yard forward sprint - 4 sets

Intensity Technique: Dynamic Effort
Dumbbell Single Arm Push Press - 3 sets of 3 reps each arm at 60% max weight

Intensity Technique: PAP Power
Alternate sets:
1A. Barbell Front Squat - 3 sets of 3 reps at 70% max weight
1B. Squat Tuck Jump - 3 sets of 5 reps

Tier 2: Assistance
Glute Ham Raise - 2 sets of 12 reps
Ring Pull-ups - 2 sets of 8–12 reps

WEEK 5
Workout #2: Pull-Up and Deadlift Power

WORKOUT NOTES

- New variations of speed development drills, plyometric exercise in PAP set, assistance exercise.

Target Area: Activation/Mobility Warm-Up
Lunge Yoga Rotations - 3 sets of 12 reps each
Foam Roll Latissimus Dorsi (Lat) Muscles - 3 sets of 30 seconds each side

Target Area: Reaction Agility (Verbal)
"W" drill on "WHISTLE" - 4 sets
Athlete changes direction *within* the "W" drill on cue from whistle

Target Area: Sprint
Circle Chase Sprints - 3 sprints in each direction
One athlete starts 3–5 yards in front of another. The other chases. On "GO," the athlete has to slap/catch the athlete in front. Use a smaller, tighter circle than previous.

Intensity Technique: PAP Power
Alternate sets:
1A. Pull-Up/Chin-Up - 3 sets of 5 reps
1B. Medicine Ball Slam - 3 sets of 5 reps

Intensity Technique: Dynamic Effort
Trap Bar Deadlift - 3 sets of 3 reps at 60% max weight

Tier 2: Assistance
Slider Single Leg Curl - 2 sets of 8 reps per leg
Ring PAUSE Push-up - 2 sets of 8–12 reps
Pause for 3 seconds at the bottom of each push-up and then *explosively* push upwards to finish the rep.

WEEK 5
Workout #3: "Fun" Friday

WORKOUT NOTES

- New variations of speed development drills and assistance exercise.
- Bicep Blaster Super Sets removed to allow more time for Medicine Ball Tennis.

OFF-SEASON II (FALL)

VARSITY LEVEL

Target Area: Activation/Mobility Warm-Up
Band Pull-Aparts - 3 sets of 25 reps
Yoga Push-Up - 3 sets of 10 reps

Target Area: Sprint
Flying 20's - 4 sets
Build up speed to a 20-yard full effort sprint

Target Area: Change of Direction
Box Depth Drop to Base Steal Sprint - 4 total sprints
Drop off a box (18–36 inches tall) and immediately sprint 10 yards, mimicking
   stealing a base.

"Big 5" Strength
Dumbbell Single Arm Bench Press
Set 1: 5 reps each arm at 45% max weight
Set 2: 5 reps each arm at 55% max weight
Set 3: 5 reps each arm at 65% max weight
Set 4: 5 reps each arm at 75% max weight

Tier 2: Assistance
Kettlebell or Dumbbell Single Leg Deadlift - 2 sets of 8 reps each leg
Dumbbell "Fat Gripz" Farmer Walk - 2 sets of 40 yards
Add "Fat Gripz" if possible

"Fun" Friday Conditioning Game
Medicine Ball Tennis

WEEK 6
Workout #1: Vertical Power

WORKOUT NOTES

- More volume (reps and sets) in the weight room

Target Area: Activation/Mobility Warm-Up
PVC or Barbell Overhead Squat - 3 sets of 5 reps with 3 second pause
Dumbbell "T" Raise (Rear Delt Raise) - 3 sets of 12 reps

Target Area: Acceleration
Sled Push Sprint (10–30% of body weight) - 6 sets of 20 yards

Target Area: Reaction Agility (Visual)
Partner 5-yard Backpedal Sprint to 5-yard Forward Sprint - 4 sets

Intensity Technique: Dynamic Effort
Dumbbell Single Arm Push Press - 4 sets of 3 reps each arm at 60% max weight

Intensity Technique: PAP Power
Alternate sets:
1A. Barbell Front Squat - 4 sets of 3 reps at 70% max weight
1B. Squat Tuck Jump - 4 sets of 3 reps

Tier 2: Assistance
Glute Ham Raise - 3 sets of 12 reps
Ring Pull-ups - 3 sets of 8–12 reps

WEEK 6
Workout #2: Pull-Up and Deadlift Power

WORKOUT NOTES

- More volume (reps and sets) in the weight room

VARSITY LEVEL   OFF-SEASON II (FALL)

Target Area: Activation/Mobility Warm-Up
Lunge Yoga Rotations - 3 sets of 12 reps each
Foam Roll Latissimus Dorsi (Lat) Muscles - 3 sets of 30 seconds each side

Target Area: Reaction Agility (Verbal)
"W" drill on "WHISTLE" - 4 sets
Athlete changes direction *within* the "W" drill on cue from whistle

Target Area: Sprint
Circle Chase Sprints - 3 sprints in each direction
One athlete starts 3–5 yards in front of another, the other chases. On "GO," the athlete has to slap/catch the athlete in front. Use a smaller, tighter circle than previous.

Intensity Technique: PAP Power
Alternate sets:
1A. Pull-Up/Chin-Up - 4 sets of 5 reps
1B. Medicine Ball Slam - 4 sets of 5 reps

Intensity Technique: Dynamic Effort
Trap Bar Deadlift - 4 sets of 3 reps at 60% max weight

Tier 2: Assistance
Slider Single Leg Curl - 2 sets of 8 reps per leg
Ring PAUSE Push-up - 2 sets of 8–12 reps
Pause for 3 seconds at the bottom of each push-up and then *explosively* push upwards to finish the rep.

WEEK 6
Workout #3: "Fun" Friday

WORKOUT NOTES

- More volume (reps and sets) in the weight room

Target Area: Activation/Mobility Warm-Up
Band Pull-Aparts - 3 sets of 25 reps
Yoga Push-Up - 3 sets of 10 reps

Target Area: Sprint
Flying 20's - 4 sets
Build up speed to a 20-yard full effort sprint

Target Area: Change of Direction
Box Depth Drop to Base steal Sprint - 4 total sprints
    Drop off a box (18–36 inches tall) and immediately sprint 10 yards, mimicking
        stealing a base.

"Big 5" Strength
Dumbbell Single Arm Bench Press
Set 1: 5 reps each arm at 45% max weight
Set 2: 8 reps each arm at 55% max weight
Set 3: 8 reps each arm at 65% max weight
Set 4: 8 reps each arm at 75% max weight

Tier 2: Assistance
Kettlebell or Dumbbell Single Leg Deadlift - 3 sets of 8 reps each leg
Dumbbell "Fat Gripz" Farmer Walk - 3 sets of 40 yards
Add "Fat Gripz" if possible

"Fun" Friday Conditioning Game
Medicine Ball Tennis

WEEK 7
Workout #1: Vertical Power

WORKOUT NOTES

- More volume (reps and sets) for the speed drills

Target Area: Activation/Mobility Warm-Up
PVC or Barbell Overhead Squat - 3 sets of 5 reps with 3 second pause
Dumbbell "T" Raise (Rear Delt Raise) - 3 sets of 12 reps

Target Area: Acceleration
Sled Push Sprint (10–30% of body weight) - 8 sets of 20 yards

Target Area: Reaction Agility (Visual)
Partner 5-yard Backpedal Sprint to 5-yard Forward Sprint - 6 sets

Intensity Technique: Dynamic Effort
Dumbbell Single Arm Push Press - 4 sets of 3 reps each arm at 60% max weight

Intensity Technique: PAP Power
Alternate sets:
1A. Barbell Front Squat - 4 sets of 3 reps at 70% max weight
1B. Squat Tuck Jump - 4 sets of 3 reps

Tier 2: Assistance
Glute Ham Raise - 3 sets of 12 reps
Ring Pull-ups - 3 sets of 8–12 reps

WEEK 7
Workout #2: Pull-Up and Deadlift Power

WORKOUT NOTES

- More volume (reps and sets) in the weight room

Target Area: Activation/Mobility Warm-Up
Lunge Yoga Rotations - 3 sets of 12 reps each
Foam Roll Latissimus Dorsi (Lat) Muscles - 3 sets of 30 seconds each side

Target Area: Reaction Agility (Verbal)
"W" drill on "WHISTLE" - 6 sets
Athlete changes direction *within* the "W" drill on cue from whistle

Target Area: Sprint
Circle Chase Sprints - 5 sprints in each direction
One athlete starts 3–5 yards in front of another. The other chases. On "GO," the athlete has to slap/catch the athlete in front. Use a smaller, tighter circle than previous.

Intensity Technique: PAP Power
Alternate sets:
1A. Pull-Up/Chin-Up - 4 sets of 5 reps
1B. Medicine Ball Slam - 4 sets of 5 reps

Intensity Technique: Dynamic Effort
Trap Bar Deadlift - 4 sets of 3 reps at 60% max weight

Tier 2: Assistance
Slider Single Leg Curl - 2 sets of 8 reps per leg
Ring PAUSE Push-up - 2 sets of 8–12 reps
Pause for 3 seconds at the bottom of each push-up and then *explosively* push upwards to finish the rep.

WEEK 7
Workout #3: "Fun" Friday

WORKOUT NOTES

- More volume (reps and sets) in the weight room

OFF-SEASON II (FALL)

VARSITY LEVEL

Target Area: Activation/Mobility Warm-Up
Band Pull-Aparts - 3 sets of 25 reps
Yoga Push-Up - 3 sets of 10 reps

Target Area: Sprint
Flying 20's - 6 sets
Build up speed to a 20-yard full effort sprint

Target Area: Change of Direction
Box Depth Drop to Base steal Sprint - 8 total sprints
Drop off a box (18–36 inches tall) and immediately sprint 10 yards mimicking
    stealing a base.

"Big 5" Strength
Dumbbell Single Arm Bench Press
Set 1: 5 reps each arm at 45% max weight
Set 2: 8 reps each arm at 55% max weight
Set 3: 8 reps each arm at 65% max weight
Set 4: 8 reps each arm at 75% max weight

Tier 2: Assistance
Kettlebell or Dumbbell Single Leg Deadlift - 3 sets of 8 reps each leg
Dumbbell "Fat Gripz" Farmer Walk - 3 sets of 40 yards
Add "Fat Gripz" if possible

"Fun" Friday Conditioning Game
Medicine Ball Tennis

WEEK 8
Workout #1: Vertical Power

WORKOUT NOTES

- Focus on crushing it in the weight room this week!

Target Area: Activation/Mobility Warm-Up
PVC or Barbell Overhead Squat - 3 sets of 5 reps with 3 second pause
Dumbbell "T" Raise (Rear Delt Raise) - 3 sets of 12 reps

Target Area: Acceleration
Sled Push Sprint (10–30% of body weight) - 8 sets of 20 yards

Target Area: Reaction Agility (Visual)
Partner 5-yard backpedal sprint to 5-yard forward sprint - 6 sets

Intensity Technique: Dynamic Effort
Dumbbell Single Arm Push Press - 4 sets of 3 reps each arm at 60% max weight

Intensity Technique: PAP Power
Alternate sets:
1A. Barbell Front Squat - 4 sets of 3 reps at 70% max weight
1B. Squat Tuck Jump - 4 sets of 3 reps

Tier 2: Assistance
Glute Ham Raise - 3 sets of 12 reps
Ring Pull-ups - 3 sets of 8–12 reps

WEEK 8
Workout #2: Pull-Up and Deadlift Power

WORKOUT NOTES

- Focus on crushing it in the weight room this week!

Target Area: Activation/Mobility Warm-Up
Lunge Yoga Rotations - 3 sets of 12 reps each
Foam Roll Latissimus Dorsi (Lat) Muscles - 3 sets of 30 seconds each side

Target Area: Reaction Agility (Verbal)
"W" drill on "WHISTLE" - 6 sets
Athlete changes direction *within* the "W" drill on cue from whistle

Target Area: Sprint
Circle Chase Sprints - 5 sprints in each direction
One athlete starts 3–5 yards in front of another. The other chases. On "GO," the
  athlete has to slap/catch the athlete in front. Use a smaller, tighter circle than
  previous.

Intensity Technique: PAP Power
Alternate sets:
1A. Pull-Up/Chin-Up - 4 sets of 5 reps
1B. Medicine Ball Slam - 4 sets of 5 reps

Intensity Technique: Dynamic Effort
Trap Bar Deadlift - 4 sets of 3 reps at 60% max weight

Tier 2: Assistance
Slider Single Leg Curl - 2 sets of 8 reps per leg
Ring PAUSE Push-up - 2 sets of 8–12 reps
Pause for 3 seconds at the bottom of each push-up and then *explosively* push
  upwards to finish the rep.

OFF-SEASON II (FALL)

VARSITY LEVEL

WEEK 8
Workout #3: "Fun" Friday

WORKOUT NOTES

- Focus on crushing it in the weight room this week!

Target Area: Activation/Mobility Warm-Up
Band Pull-Aparts - 3 sets of 25 reps
Yoga Push-Up - 3 sets of 10 reps

Target Area: Sprint
Flying 20's - 6 sets
Build up speed to a 20-yard full effort sprint

Target Area: Change of Direction
Box Depth Drop to Base Steal Sprint - 8 total sprints
Drop off a box (18–36 inches tall) and immediately sprint 10 yards mimicking
    stealing a base.

"Big 5" Strength
Dumbbell Single Arm Bench Press
Set 1: 5 reps each arm at 45% max weight
Set 2: 8 reps each arm at 55% max weight
Set 3: 8 reps each arm at 65% max weight
Set 4: 8 reps each arm at 75% max weight

Tier 2: Assistance
Kettlebell or Dumbbell Single Leg Deadlift - 3 sets of 8 reps each leg
Dumbbell "Fat Gripz" Farmer Walk - 3 sets of 40 yards
Add "Fat Gripz" if possible

"Fun" Friday Conditioning Game
Medicine Ball Tennis

PRE-SEASON I (WINTER)

Beginning with a transition week at the start of the winter season, players are given time to learn the new movements of this phase and build up slowly after their much-needed downtime after fall ball.

This program utilizes three full body lifts and two days of speed development work per week in an effort to have you at your physical best for the start of the spring season. We also anticipate more time in the weight room (compared to the fall program) because the fall baseball season is over. We rotate workouts in the weight room that focus on power development—namely PAP sets and dynamic effort sets—and good old-fashioned strength work. The speed days focus on acceleration, change of direction, reaction agility, and team competition drills. I program Medicine Ball Tennis on lift days, but ultimately, play whenever you can.

This phase includes all "Big 5" exercises along with variations, and all Tier 2 and Tier 3 core lift movements. It also includes additional posterior chain work (glute, hamstring, back, and upper back) to balance all the pushing muscles used, in an effort to stay injury-free.

Program Breakdown

Monday: Strength	Tuesday: Speed	Wednesday: Strength	Thursday: Speed	Friday: Strength
Target Area: Dynamic Warm-Up	**Target Area:** Dynamic Warm-Up	**Target Area:** Dynamic Warm-Up	**Target Area:** Dynamic Warm-Up	**Target Area:** Dynamic Warm-Up
Target Area: **Acceleration** Heavy Sled Push **Intensity** **Technique:** **PAP Power** 1A. Shoulder Press 1B. Medicine Ball Squat Press Throw **Tier 2:** Carry **Tier 3:** **Posterior** **Chain** Lower	**Target Area:** Mobility **Tier 2:** **Rotation** Medicine Ball Throw **Target** **Area: Speed** **Development** *Acceleration *Change of Direction *Sprint (Race and Chase) Cool down stretch/ massage	**Intensity** **Technique:** **PAP Power** 1A. Back Squat 1B. Vertical Jump **Mechanical** **Drop Set** Pull-Up or Chin-Up TRX or Ring Row **Tier 2: Lunge** 747 **Tier 3:** **Posterior** **Chain** Upper	**Target Area:** Mobility **Tier 2: Jump** Lateral Plyometrics **Target** **Area: Speed** **Development** *Reaction Agility *Acceleration *Sprint (Race and Chase) Cool down stretch/ massage	**Intensity** **Technique:** **Dynamic** **Effort** Speed Bench Press **Intensity** **Technique:** **PAP Power** 1A. Trap Bar Jump Shrug 1B. Horizontal Jump **Tier 3:** **Posterior** **Chain** Upper **Tier 3:** **Posterior** **Chain** Lower

PROGRAM NOTES

- Alternate speed workouts with lift workouts. For example, lift Monday/Wednesday/Friday and perform speed drills on Tuesday/Thursday.

- The dynamic warm-up is too long to include with the daily workouts. Please refer to Appendix A: Speed Development Playbook on GetFitNow.com.

- Set up the drills as stations after the dynamic warm-up and mobility movements as space and equipment dictates.

- General reps and sets are given, but only a coach running the workout can accurately assign reps and sets based on an athlete's conditioning levels and general pace of the workout.

WEEK 1
Workout #1: Transition Week

Target Area: Mobility Warm-Up
Single Leg Glute Bridge (foot elevated on bench) - 1 set of 6 reps per leg
Yoga Push-Ups - 1 set of 10 reps
PVC Bench Thoracic Extension - 1 set of 5 deep breaths

Tier 1: Strength
Sled Push - 4 sets of 10 yards
    Push a sled equal to half your body weight.

Assistance
Trap Bar Farmers Walks - 2 sets of 20–30 yards
3D Barbell Hip Thrust (mini band or slingshot around the knees) - 2 sets of 8 reps

Recovery
Finish each day with a 10 minute foam roll massage

WEEK 1
Workout #2: Transition Week

Target Area: Mobility Warm-Up
PVC or Empty Barbell Overhead Squat - 1 set of 10 reps
Walking Lunge with Rotation - 1 set of 10 reps per leg
Band Overhead Squat Pattern - 1 set of 10 reps

Tier 1: Strength
Barbell Back Squat - 2 sets of 5 reps
    Use 50% of max weight and focus on full depth and technique

Intensity Technique: Mechanical Drop Set
Perform 2 sets each of:
1A. Pull-Up or Chin-Up - 10 reps
1B. TRX or Ring Row - 10 reps

Assistance
Dumbbell Bulgarian Squat 747 - 1 set
Dumbbell Supported Row - 2 sets of 12 reps

Recovery
Finish each day with a 10 minute foam roll massage

VARSITY LEVEL   PRE-SEASON I (WINTER)

WEEK 1
Workout #3: Transition Week

Target Area: Mobility Warm-Up
Band Pull-Aparts - 1 set of 25 reps
Medicine Ball Thoracic Extension - 1 set of 5 deep breaths
Dumbbell "T" Balance - 1 set of 8 reps per leg

Tier 1: Power
Trap Bar Jump Shrug - 2 sets of 5 reps
    Max weight used should be 30–50% of max weight.

Assistance
Cable or Band Face Pull - 2 sets of 15 reps
TRX or Physioball Leg Curl - 2 sets of 15 reps

Recovery
Finish each day with a 10 minute foam roll massage

WEEK 2
Workout #1: Sled Strength and Vertical Power

WORKOUT NOTES

- Rest as necessary to be at full strength for each set of heavy sled push.

Target Area: Dynamic Warm-Up
Single Leg Glute Bridge (foot elevated on bench) - 3 sets of 12 reps per leg
Yoga Push-Ups - 3 sets of 10 reps
PVC Bench Thoracic Extension - 3 sets of 5 deep breaths

Tier 1: Strength
Heavy Sled Push - 4 sets of 10–20 yards
    Push a sled equal to your body weight.

Intensity Technique: PAP Power
Alternate sets:
1A. Dumbbell Shoulder Press - 4 sets of 3 reps at 65% max weight
1B. Medicine Ball Squat Press Throw - 4 sets of 5 reps

Tier 2: Carry
Trap Bar Farmers Walks - 4 sets of 20–30 yards

Tier 3: Posterior Chain (Lower)
3D Barbell Hip Thrust (mini band or slingshot around the knees) - 2 sets of
    15 reps

Optional Conditioning Game
Medicine Ball Tennis

WEEK 2
Workout #2: Speed Day

WORKOUT NOTES

- See Appendix A: Speed Development Playbook on GetFitNow.com for a full dynamic warm-up.
- Athletes should be in small groups to race for Speed Development (Change of Direction) drills.

Target Area: Dynamic Warm-Up

Target Area: Mobility
Lunge Yoga Rotation - 2 sets of 10 reps per side
Linear Leg Swings - 2 sets of 10 reps per side
    Cue "TOES UP!"
Lateral Leg Swings - 2 sets of 10 reps per side
    Cue "TOES UP!"
Active Prehab: Ankle Mobility - 2 sets of 10 reps per side
    Hold the top of your yoga push-up position and alternate driving your knees forward to mobilize your ankles.

Tier 2: Rotation
Partner Medicine Ball Rotation Throws - 3 sets of 5 reps
    Stand as far as possible from your partner to catch the ball in the air. Take a step further away from each other each rep you catch. Take a step closer to each other if you drop the ball.

Target Area: Speed Development (Acceleration)
Light Sled Push, Hill Sprints, or Stadium Stairs - 6 sets of 10 yards
    Use 25–50% of Monday's sled weight.

Target Area: Speed Development (Change of Direction)
3-cone Drill - 6 sets
60-yard Shuttle Runs - 4 sets
    5 yards out and back, 10 yards out and back, 15 yards out and back counts as 1 set.

Target Area: Speed Development (Sprint)
Swim Noodle Chase Drill - 10 sets of 30 yards
>One athlete starts 3–5 yards in front of another. The other chases, holding a swim noodle. On "GO," the athlete with the swim noodle has to slap/catch the athlete in front before he reaches 30 yards.

Cool down stretch and foam roll massage

WEEK 2
Workout #3: PAP Squat Day

WORKOUT NOTES

- Rest as necessary to be at full strength for each set of back squat.
- If you cannot perform a full pull-up or chin-up, please substitute your pull-up/chin-up progression exercise into the mechanical drop set.
- Perform weighted pull-ups after you can do 4 sets of 10 reps of body weight.

Target Area: Dynamic Warm-Up
PVC or Empty Barbell Overhead Squat - 3 sets of 10 reps
Walking Lunge with Rotation - 3 sets of 10 reps each leg
Band Overhead Squat Pattern - 3 sets of 10 reps

Intensity Technique: PAP Power
Alternate sets:
1A. Barbell Back Squat - 4 sets of 3 reps at 65% max weight
1B. Rotational Squat Jump - 4 sets of 3 reps each direction
Jump vertically and land in a 90-degree turn. Quickly jump again and land in your original direction. This constitutes one rep.

Mechanical Drop Set
2A. Pull-Up or Chin-Up - 4 sets of 10 reps
2B. TRX or Ring Row - 4 sets of AMRAP

Tier 2: Lunge
Dumbbell Bulgarian Squat 747 - 2 sets

Tier 3: Posterior Chain (Upper)
Dumbbell Supported Row - 2 sets of 12 reps

Optional Conditioning Game
Medicine Ball Tennis

WEEK 2
Workout #4: Speed Day

WORKOUT NOTES

- See Appendix A: Development Playbook on GetFitNow.com Playbook for a full dynamic warm-up.
- Athletes should be in small groups to race for Speed Development (Change of Direction) drills.

Target Area: Dynamic Warm-Up

Target Area: Mobility
Lunge Yoga Rotation - 2 sets of 10 reps per side
Linear Leg Swings - 2 sets of 10 reps per side
    Cue "TOES UP!"
Lateral Leg Swings - 2 sets of 10 reps per side
    Cue "TOES UP!"
Active Prehab: Ankle Mobility - 2 sets of 10 reps per side
    Hold the top of your yoga push-up position and alternate driving your knees forward to mobilize your ankles.

Tier 2: Jump (Lateral Plyometrics)
Inside Edge Lateral Line Bound with Stabilization - 3 sets of 8 reps per leg
    Hop off the inside edge of your foot from left to right/right to left along the lines of the track at a 45-degree angle. Stick each landing.

Target Area: Speed Development (Reaction Agility)
(Cognitive) Push-Ups - 8 sets
    Start 20-yard sprints on "RED"

Target Area: Speed Development (Acceleration)
Stadium Stairs (two stairs at a time) - 4–6 sets of 10 steps per leg

Target Area: Speed Development (Sprint)
20-yard Angled Swim Noodle Chase Drill
    One athlete starts 3–5 yards in front of another. The other chases, holding a swim noodle. On "GO," the athlete with the swim noodle has to slap/catch the athlete in front before he reaches 30 yards.
Cool down stretch and foam roll massage

WEEK 2
Workout #5: Dynamic Effort Bench Day

WORKOUT NOTES

- Rest as needed to be at full strength for each dynamic effort bench set. Use a SWIS or Neutral Grip Barbell with chains or bands if available.
- Perform Dumbbell Speed Bench Press with fast and powerful up and down reps.
- Use about 50–60% of your trap bar deadlift max for trap bar jump shrug sets.

Target Area: Dynamic Warm-Up
Band Pull-Aparts - 3 sets of 25 reps
Medicine Ball Thoracic Extension - 3 sets of 5 deep breaths
Dumbbell "T" Balance - 3 sets of 8 reps per leg

Intensity Technique: Dynamic Effort
Dumbbell Speed Bench Press - 8 sets of 3 reps at 55% max weight

Intensity Technique: PAP Power
Alternate sets:
1A. Trap Bar Jump Shrug - 4 sets of 3 reps at 65% max weight
1B. Broad Jump DOUBLES - 4 sets of 3 reps
    DOUBLES = 2 consecutive broad jumps

Tier 3: Posterior Chain (Upper)
Cable or Band Face Pull - 2 sets of 15 reps

Tier 3: Posterior Chain (Lower)
TRX or Physioball Leg Curl - 2 sets of 15 reps

Optional Conditioning Game
Medicine Ball Tennis

WEEK 3
Workout #1: Sled Strength and Vertical Power

WORKOUT NOTES
- More sets added to the heavy sled push
- Add weight to the dumbbell shoulder press

Target Area: Dynamic Warm-Up
Single Leg Glute Bridge (foot elevated on bench) - 3 sets of 12 reps per leg
Yoga Push-Ups - 3 sets of 10 reps
PVC Bench Thoracic Extension - 3 sets of 5 deep breaths

Tier 1: Strength
Heavy Sled Push - 6 sets of 10–20 yards
    Push a sled equal to your body weight.

Intensity Technique: PAP Power
Alternate sets:
1A. Dumbbell Shoulder Press - 4 sets of 3 reps at 70% max weight
1B. Medicine Ball Squat Press Throw - 4 sets of 5 reps

Tier 2: Carry
Trap Bar Farmers Walks - 4 sets of 20–30 yards

Tier 3: Posterior Chain (Lower)
3D Barbell Hip Thrust (mini band or slingshot around the knees) - 2 sets of
    15 reps

Optional Conditioning Game
Medicine Ball Tennis

WEEK 3
Workout #2: Speed Day

WORKOUT NOTES

- See Appendix A: Speed Development Playbook on GetFitNow.com for a full dynamic warm-up.
- New change of direction exercise
- Athletes should be in small groups to race for Speed Development (Change of Direction) drills.

Target Area: Dynamic Warm-Up

Target Area: Mobility
Lunge Yoga Rotation - 2 sets of 10 reps per side
Linear Leg Swings - 2 sets of 10 reps per side
    Cue "TOES UP!"
Lateral Leg Swings - 2 sets of 10 reps per side
    Cue "TOES UP!"
Active Prehab: Ankle Mobility - 2 sets of 10 reps per each side
    Hold the top of your yoga push-up position and alternate your knees forward
        to mobilize your ankles.

Tier 2: Rotation
Partner Medicine Ball Rotation Throws - 3 sets of 5 reps
    Stand as far as possible from your partner to catch the ball in the air. Take a
        step further away from each other each rep you catch. Take a step closer
        to each other if you drop the ball.

Target Area: Speed Development (Acceleration)
Light Sled Push or Hill Sprints - 6 sets of 10 yards
    Use 25–50% of Monday's weight for sled.

Target Area: Speed Development (Change of Direction)
3-cone Drill - 6 sets
Pro Agility (5–10–5) - 3 sets in each direction

Target Area: Speed Development (Sprint)

Swim Noodle Chase Drill - 10 sets of 30 yards

One athlete starts 3–5 yards in front of another. The other chases, holding a swim noodle. On "GO," the athlete with the swim noodle has to slap/ catch the athlete in front before he reaches 30 yards.

Cool down stretch and foam roll massage

WEEK 3
Workout #3: PAP Squat Day

WORKOUT NOTES
- Add weight to the back squat
- Add rep speed if possible to the pull-up/chin-up.
- If the athlete cannot perform a full pull-up or chin-up, please substitute their pull-up/chin-up progression exercise into the mechanical drop set. Perform weighted pull-ups after the athlete can do 4 sets of 10 reps of body weight.

Target Area: Dynamic Warm-Up
PVC or Empty Barbell Overhead Squat - 3 sets of 10 reps
Walking Lunge with Rotation - 3 sets of 10 reps per leg
Band Overhead Squat Pattern - 3 sets of 10 reps

Intensity Technique: PAP Power
Alternate sets:
1A. Barbell Back Squat - 4 sets of 3 reps at 70% max weight
1B. Rotational Squat Jump - 4 sets of 3 reps each direction
    Jump vertically and land in a 90 degree turn. Quickly jump again and land in your original direction. That equals one rep.

Intensity Technique: Mechanical Drop Set
2A. Pull-Up or Chin-Up - 4 sets of 10 reps
2B. TRX or Ring Row - 4 sets of AMRAP

Tier 2: Lunge
Dumbbell Bulgarian Squat 747 - 2 sets

Tier 3: Posterior Chain (Upper)
Dumbbell Supported Row - 2 sets of 12 reps

Optional Conditioning Game
Medicine Ball Tennis

WEEK 3
Workout #4: Speed Day

WORKOUT NOTES

- See Appendix A: Speed Development Playbook on GetFitNow.com for a full dynamic warm-up.
- New reaction agility exercise
- Athletes should be in small groups to race for Speed Development (Change of Direction) drills.

Target Area: Dynamic Warm-Up

Target Area: Mobility
Lunge Yoga Rotation - 2 sets of 10 reps per side
Linear Leg Swings - 2 sets of 10 reps per side
    Cue "TOES UP!"
Lateral Leg Swings - 2 sets of 10 reps per side
    Cue "TOES UP!"
Active Prehab: Ankle Mobility - 2 sets of 10 reps per side
    Hold the top of your yoga push-up position and alternate your knees forward to mobilize your ankles.

Tier 2: Jump (Lateral Plyometrics)
Inside Edge Lateral Line Bound with Stabilization - 3 sets of 8 reps per leg
    Hop off the inside edge of your foot, going from left to right/right to left along the lines of the track at a 45-degree angle. Stick each landing.

Target Area: Speed Development (Reaction Agility)
(Visual) Competition Push-Up Sprints - 8 sets
    Start 20-yard sprints on the first movement of the athlete designated as leader.

Target Area: Speed Development (Acceleration)
Stadium Stairs (two stairs at a time) - 4–6 sets of 10 steps each leg

Target Area: Speed Development (Sprint)
20-yard Angled Swim Noodle Chase Drill
> One athlete starts 3–5 yards in front of the other and at a 45-degree angle. The other athlete is holding a swim noodle. On "GO," the athlete with the swim noodle has to slap/catch the athlete in front before he reaches 30 yards.

Cool down stretch and foam roll massage

WEEK 3
Workout #5: Dynamic Effort Bench Day

WORKOUT NOTES

- Rest as needed to be at full strength for each dynamic effort bench set. Use a SWIS or Neutral Grip Barbell with chains or bands if available.
- Perform Dumbbell Speed Bench Press with fast and powerful up and down reps.
- Progress to 5 reps per set on the Trap Bar Jump Shrug.

Target Area: Dynamic Warm-Up
Band Pull-Aparts - 3 sets of 25 reps
Medicine Ball Thoracic Extension - 3 sets of 5 deep breaths
Dumbbell "T" Balance - 3 sets of 8 reps per leg

Intensity Technique: Dynamic Effort
Dumbbell SPEED Bench Press - 6 sets of 3 reps at 60% max weight

Intensity Technique: PAP Power
Alternate sets:
1A. Trap Bar Jump Shrug - 4 sets of 5 reps at 50–60% max weight
1B. Broad Jump DOUBLES - 4 sets of 3 reps
      DOUBLES = 2 consecutive broad jumps

Tier 3: Posterior Chain (Upper)
Cable or Band Face Pull - 2 sets of 15 reps

Tier 3: Posterior Chain (Lower)
TRX or Physioball Leg Curl - 2 sets of 15 reps

Optional Conditioning Game
Medicine Ball Tennis

WEEK 4
Workout #1: Sled Strength and Vertical Power

WORKOUT NOTES

- Add volume (reps and sets) to the assistance work this week.

Target Area: Dynamic Warm-Up
Single Leg Glute Bridge (foot elevated on bench) - 3 sets of 12 reps per leg
Yoga Push-Ups - 3 sets of 10 reps
PVC Bench Thoracic Extension - 3 sets of 5 deep breaths

Tier 1: Strength
Heavy Sled Push - 6 sets of 10-20 yards
    Push a sled equal to your body weight.

Intensity Technique: PAP Power
Alternate sets:
1A. Dumbbell Shoulder Press - 4 sets of 3 reps at 70% max weight
1B. Medicine Ball Squat Press Throw - 4 sets of 5 reps

Tier 2: Carry
Trap Bar Farmers Walks - 4 sets of 30–40 yards

Tier 3: Posterior Chain (Lower)
3D Barbell Hip Thrust (mini band or slingshot around the knees) - 4 sets of 8 reps

Optional Conditioning Game
Medicine Ball Tennis

WEEK 4
Workout #2: Speed Day

WORKOUT NOTES

- See Appendix A: Speed Development Playbook on GetFitNow.com for a full dynamic warm-up.
- New change of direction exercise
- Athletes should be in small groups to race for Speed Development (Change of Direction) drills.

Target Area: Dynamic Warm-Up

Target Area: Mobility
Lunge Yoga Rotation - 2 sets of 10 reps per side
Linear Leg Swings - 2 sets of 10 reps per side
    Cue "TOES UP!"
Lateral Leg Swings - 2 sets of 10 reps per side
    Cue "TOES UP!"
Active Prehab: Ankle Mobility - 2 sets of 10 reps per side
    Hold the top of your yoga push-up position and alternate driving your knees
        forward to mobilize your ankles.

Tier 2: Rotation
Partner Medicine Ball Rotation Throws - 3 sets of 5 reps
    Stand as far as possible from your partner to catch the ball in the air. Take a
        step further away from each other each rep you catch. Take a step closer
        to each other if you drop the ball.

Target Area: Speed Development (Acceleration)
Light Sled Push or Hill Sprints - 6 sets of 10 yards
    Use 25–50% of Monday's sled weight.

Target Area: Speed Development (Change of Direction)
"W" Drill - 6 sets
    Set up cones in a "W" pattern, 5 yards apart. Sprint cone to cone, forwards
        and backwards, facing the same direction through the entire drill.
Pro Agility (5–10–5) - 3 sets each direction

Target Area: Speed Development (Sprint)

Swim Noodle Chase Drill - 10 sets of 30 yards

One athlete starts 3–5 yards in front of another. The other chases, holding a swim noodle. On "GO," the athlete with the swim noodle has to slap/catch the athlete in front before he reaches 30 yards.

Cool down stretch and foam roll massage

WEEK 4
Workout #3: PAP Squat Day

WORKOUT NOTES

- Add volume (reps and sets) to the assistance work this week.
- Add rep speed if possible to the pull-up/chin-up
- If you cannot perform a full pull-up or chin-up, please substitute your pull-up/chin-up progression exercise into the mechanical drop set. Perform weighted pull-ups after you can do 4 sets of 10 reps of body weight.

Target Area: Dynamic Warm-Up
PVC or Empty Barbell Overhead Squat - 3 sets of 10 reps
Walking Lunge with Rotation - 3 sets of 10 reps each leg
Band Overhead Squat Pattern - 3 sets of 10 reps

Intensity Technique: PAP Power
Alternate sets:
1A. Barbell Back Squat - 4 sets of 3 reps at 70% max weight
1B. Rotational Squat Jump - 4 sets of 3 reps each direction
    Jump vertically and land in a 90-degree turn. Quickly jump again and land in your original direction. This constitutes one rep.

Mechanical Drop Set
2A. Pull-Up or Chin-Up - 4 sets of 10 reps
2B. TRX or Ring Row - 4 sets of AMRAP

Tier 2: Lunge
Dumbbell Bulgarian Squat 747 - 3 sets of 12 reps

Tier 3: Posterior Chain (Upper)
Dumbbell Supported Row - 3 sets of 12 reps

Optional Conditioning Game
Medicine Ball Tennis

WEEK 4
Workout #4: Speed Day

WORKOUT NOTES

- See Appendix A: Speed Development Playbook on GetFitNow.com for a full dynamic warm-up.
- New reaction agility exercise
- Athletes should be in small groups to race for Speed Development (Change of Direction) drills.

Target Area: Dynamic Warm-Up

Target Area: Mobility
Lunge Yoga Rotation - 2 sets of 10 reps per side
Linear Leg Swings - 2 sets of 10 reps per side
    Cue "TOES UP!"
Lateral Leg Swings - 2 sets of 10 reps per side
    Cue "TOES UP!"
Active Prehab: Ankle Mobility - 2 sets of 10 reps per side
    Hold the top of your yoga push-up position and alternate driving your knees forward to mobilize your ankles.

Tier 2: Jump (Lateral Plyometrics)
Inside Edge Lateral Line Bound with Stabilization - 3 sets of 8 reps per leg
    Hop off the inside edge of your foot from left to right/right to left along the lines of the track at a 45-degree angle. Stick each landing.

Target Area: Speed Development (Reaction Agility)
(Verbal) Competition Half Kneeling (Lunge) Sprints - 8 sets
    Start 20-yard sprints on "GO!" or any predetermined trigger.

Target Area: Speed Development (Acceleration)
Stadium Stairs (two stairs at a time) - 4–6 sets of 10 steps per leg

Target Area: Speed Development (Sprint)
20-yard Angled Swim Noodle Chase Drill
> One athlete starts 3–5 yards in front of the other and at a 45-degree angle. The other athlete is holding a swim noodle. On "GO," the athlete with the swim noodle has to slap/catch the one in front before he reaches 30 yards.

Cool down stretch and foam roll massage

WEEK 4
Workout #5: Dynamic Effort Bench Day

WORKOUT NOTES

- Rest as needed to be at full strength for each dynamic effort bench set. Use a SWIS or Neutral Grip Barbell with chains or bands if available.
- Perform Dumbbell Speed Bench Press with fast and powerful up and down reps.
- Add volume (reps and sets) to the assistance work this week.

Target Area: Dynamic Warm-Up
Band Pull-Aparts - 3 sets of 25 reps
Medicine Ball Thoracic Extension - 3 sets of 5 deep breaths
Dumbbell "T" Balance - 3 sets of 8 reps per leg

Intensity Technique: Dynamic Effort
Dumbbell SPEED Bench Press - 6 sets of 3 reps at 60% max weight

Intensity Technique: PAP Power
Alternate sets:
1A. Trap Bar Jump Shrug - 4 sets of 5 reps at 50–60% max weight
1B. Broad Jump DOUBLES - 4 sets of 3 reps
    DOUBLES = 2 consecutive broad jumps

Tier 3: Posterior Chain (Upper)
Cable or Band Face Pull - 3 sets of 15 reps

Tier 3: Posterior Chain (Lower)
TRX or Physioball Leg Curl - 3 sets of 15 reps

Optional Conditioning Game
Medicine Ball Tennis

PRE-SEASON II (WINTER)

S tarting with a transition week to refresh from the first four weeks of work and to learn the new exercises for this 4-week phase, the second half of the pre-season program rotates the exercises used for PAP power, dynamic effort, and strength and introduces new speed drills. We also incorporate simple progressions for one of the assistance exercises each workout.

This phase also introduces two new protocols, rest/pause and PSD sets.

Rest/pause sets are, in a word, brutal. They call for shorter rest periods in between traditional strength building sets. Traditional strength training calls for 60 seconds to 2 minutes of rest between sets, where rest/pause sets call for 15–30 seconds (or 3–5 deep breaths) between sets. The goal for rest/pause sets is to finish more reps for an exercise where you otherwise could not. For this phase, I program rest/pause pull-ups or chin-ups, as this body weight exercise is perfect for pushing your physical limits safely.

PSD sets are equally brutal. PSD sets utilize the old school bodybuilding techniques of a pre-exhaust set, a strength set, and a mechanical drop set, programmed in a circuit format.

An example of a PSD set example for working the shoulders would be:

1A. Dumbbell Lateral Raise for 8–12 reps with 25 lbs.
Looking for a moderate (but not to failure) pump in the shoulders.
1B. Dumbbell Shoulder Press for 6–8 reps with 50 lbs.
Max effort strength exercise (to near failure)
1C. Dumbbell Lateral Raise for 10+ reps with 20 lbs.
5–10 lbs. lighter than the 1A set, taken to failure

Program Breakdown

Monday: Strength	Tuesday: Speed	Wednesday: Strength	Thursday: Speed	Friday: Strength
Target Area: Dynamic Warm-Up	**Target Area:** Dynamic Warm-Up	**Target Area:** Dynamic Warm-Up	**Target Area:** Dynamic Warm-Up	**Target Area:** Dynamic Warm-Up
Intensity Technique: PAP Power 1A. Dumbbell Incline Bench Press 1B. Plyo Push-Up	**Target Area:** Mobility	**Intensity Technique: PAP Power** 1A. Heavy Sled Push 1B. Broad Jump	**Target Area:** Mobility	**Intensity Technique: Dynamic Effort** Barbell Front Pause Squat
Tier 1: Olympic Strength Dumbbell Single Arm Snatch	**Tier 2: Rotation** Medicine Ball Throw **Target Area: Speed Development** *Over Speed Sprints *Acceleration *Change of Direction	**Intensity Technique: Rest/Pause** Pull-Up or Chin-Up	**Tier 2: Jump** Lateral Plyometrics **Target Area: Speed Development** *Reaction Agility *Acceleration *Sprint (Race and Chase)	**Intensity Technique: PSD** Shoulders
Tier 2: Carry **Tier 3: Posterior Chain** Lower	Cool down stretch/ massage	**Tier 2: Lunge** Lateral **Tier 3: Posterior Chain** Upper	Cool down stretch/ massage	**Tier 3: Posterior Chain** Upper **Tier 3: Posterior Chain** Lower

PROGRAM NOTES

- The dynamic warm-up is too long to include with each of the daily workouts. Please refer to Appendix A: Speed Development Playbook on GetFitNow.com.

- Set the drills up as stations after the dynamic warm-up and mobility movements as space and equipment dictates.

- General reps and sets are given, but only a coach running the workout can accurately assign reps and sets based on their athlete's conditioning levels and general pace of the workout.

- Acceleration work now focuses on lighter loads to build more speed and strength.

- Program now includes over speed drills. The key is to slightly push your limits without a breakdown in your running technique. If you force your body to move too fast, your feet will hit in front of your body, inhibiting max speed.

- As always, continue the Medicine Ball Tennis when possible.

WEEK 5
Workout #1: Transition Week

Target Area: Mobility Warm-Up
Single Leg Glute Bridge (foot elevated on bench) - 1 set of 6 reps per leg
Yoga Push-Ups - 1 set of 10 reps
PVC Bench Thoracic Extension - 1 set of 5 deep breaths

Tier 1: Strength
Dumbbell Incline Bench Press - 2 sets of 5 reps

Tier 1: Olympic Strength (Practice)
Dumbbell Single Arm Snatch - 3 sets of 5 reps per arm
    Use lighter weights to help focus on technique.

Assistance
Dumbbell Single Arm Farmers Walks - 2 sets of 20–30 yards per side
3D Barbell Hip Thrust (mini band or slingshot around the knees) - 2 sets of 8 reps

Recovery
Finish each day with 10 minutes foam roll massage

WEEK 5
Workout #2: Transition Week

Target Area: Mobility Warm-Up
PVC or Empty Barbell Overhead Squat - 1 set of 10 reps
Walking Lunge with Rotation - 1 set of 10 reps per leg
Band Overhead Squat Pattern - 1 set of 10 reps

Tier 1: Strength
Sled Push - 4 sets of 10 yards
    Push a sled equal to half your body weight.

Rest/Pause
Pull-Up or Chin-Up - 2 sets
    Limit your reps to about 50% of your max reps.

Assistance
Dumbbell Lateral Lunge - 1 set of 8 reps per side
Dumbbell Supported Row - 2 sets of 12 reps

Recovery
Finish each day with 10 minutes foam roll massage

WEEK 5
Workout #3: Transition Week

Target Area: Mobility Warm-Up
Band Pull-Aparts - 1 set of 25 reps
Medicine Ball Thoracic Extension - 1 set of 5 deep breaths
Dumbbell "T" Balance - 1 set of 8 reps per leg

Tier 1: Power
Barbell Front Pause Front - 2 sets of 5 reps
    Weight used should be 50% of max to practice good depth and pause.

Assistance
Cable or Band Face Pull - 2 sets of 15 reps
TRX or Physioball Single Leg Curl - 2 sets of 10 reps per leg

Recovery
Finish each day with 10 minutes foam roll massage

WEEK 6
Workout #1: Bench and Jump Power Day

WORKOUT NOTES

- Rest as necessary to be at full strength for each set of incline bench press.

Target Area: Dynamic Warm-Up
Single Leg Glute Bridge (foot elevated on bench) - 3 sets of 12 reps per leg
Yoga Push-Ups - 3 sets of 10 reps
PVC Bench Thoracic Extension - 3 sets of 5 deep breaths

Intensity Technique: PAP Power
Alternate sets:
1A. Dumbbell Incline Bench Press - 3 sets of 3 reps at 65% max weight
1B. Plyo (clap) Push-Ups - 3 sets of 5 reps

Tier 1: Olympic Strength
Dumbbell Single Arm Snatch - 3 sets of 5 reps per arm

Tier 2: Carry
Dumbbell Single Arm Farmers Walks - 2 sets of 20–30 yards per side

Tier 3: Posterior Chain (Lower)
3D Barbell Hip Thrust (mini band or slingshot around the knees) - 2 sets of
15 reps

WEEK 6
Workout #2: Speed Day

WORKOUT NOTES

- See Appendix A: Speed Development Playbook on GetFitNow.com for a full dynamic warm-up.
- For the over speed drill, the band, bungee or tow strap should only pull/assist/force the athlete to run faster 5–10% for the first 5–10 yards or 3–5 strides. After that, release the athlete and allow them to finish the sprint.
- Athletes should be in small groups to race for Speed Development (Change of Direction) drills.

Target Area: Dynamic Warm-Up

Target Area: Mobility
Lunge Yoga Rotation - 2 sets of 10 reps per side
Linear Leg Swings - 2 sets of 10 reps per side
    Cue "TOES UP!"
Lateral Leg Swings - 2 sets of 10 reps per side
    Cue "TOES UP!"
Active Prehab: Ankle Mobility - 2 sets of 10 reps per side
    Hold the top of your yoga push-up position and alternate driving your knees forward to mobilize your ankles.

Tier 2: Rotation
Partner Medicine Ball Shuffle Rotation Throws - 3 sets of 5 reps per direction
    Stand as far as possible from your partner to catch the ball in the air. Take a step further away from each other each rep you catch. Take a step closer to each other if you drop the ball.

Target Area: Speed Development (Over Speed)
Light Assist (Band, Bungee, or Tow Strap) Sprint - 4 sets of 20–30 yards

Target Area: Speed Development (Acceleration)
Moderate Sled Push - 6 sets of 30–50% of your body weight

Target Area: Speed Development (Change of Direction)
Ice Skater Jumps to Forward Sprint - 4 sets of 20 yard sprints
5-yard Backpedal Sprint to 5-yard Forward Sprint - 4 sets
Cool down stretch and foam roll massage

WEEK 6
Workout #3: PAP Sled Push Day

WORKOUT NOTES

- Rest as necessary to be at full strength for each set of sled push.
- If the athlete cannot perform a full pull-up or chin-up, please substitute their pull-up/chin-up progression exercise into the rest/pause set.
- For the rest/pause set: Performing a set at 80% max effort, followed by 3–5 deep breaths, then a second max effort set, followed by 3–5 deep breaths, and finally a third max effort set, constitutes 1 "set" of rest/pause. Each round of a rest/pause set should see diminishing rep counts as you push yourself.

Target Area: Dynamic Warm-Up
PVC or Empty Barbell Overhead Squat - 3 sets of 10 reps
Walking Lunge with Rotation - 3 sets of 10 reps per leg
Band Overhead Squat Pattern - 3 sets of 10 reps

Intensity Technique: PAP Power
Alternate sets:
1A. Heavy Sled Push (Body Weight) - 3 sets of 10 yards
1B. Broad Jump TRIPLES - 3 sets of 2 reps
    TRIPLES = 3 consecutive broad jumps

Intensity Technique: Rest/Pause
Pull-Up or Chin-Up - 2 sets

Tier 2: Lunge
Dumbbell Lateral Lunge - 2 sets of 12 reps per side

Tier 3: Posterior Chain (Upper)
Dumbbell Supported Row - 2 sets of 12 reps

WEEK 6
Workout #4: Speed Day

WORKOUT NOTES

- See Appendix A: Speed Development Playbook on GetFitNow.com for a full dynamic warm-up.
- Athletes should be in small groups to race for Speed Development (Change of Direction) drills.

Target Area: Dynamic Warm-Up

Target Area: Mobility
Lunge Yoga Rotation - 2 sets of 10 reps per side
Linear Leg Swings - 2 sets of 10 reps per side
    Cue "TOES UP!"
Lateral Leg Swings - 2 sets of 10 reps per side
    Cue "TOES UP!"
Active Prehab: Ankle Mobility - 2 sets of 10 reps per side
    Hold the top of your yoga push-up position and alternate driving your knees forward to mobilize your ankles.

Tier 2: Jump (Lateral Plyometrics)
Outside Edge (X-over) Lateral Line Bound with Stabilization - 3 sets of 8 reps per leg
    Hop off the outside edge of your foot (X-over) from left to right/right to left along the lines of the track at a 45-degree angle. Stick each landing.

Target Area: Speed Development (Reaction Agility)
(Cognitive) Pro Agility (5–10–5) Drill - 6 sets
    Sprint left on "EVEN NUMBER" and sprint right on "ODD NUMBER"

Target Area: Speed Development (Acceleration)
Resisted (Band or Bungee) High Knee Sprint - 6 sets of 10 yards

Target Area: Speed Development (Sprint)
Flying 20's - 8 sets
    Build up your speed to a 20-yard full effort sprint
Cool down stretch and foam roll massage

WEEK 6
Workout #5: Dynamic Effort Front Squat Day

WORKOUT NOTES

- Rest as needed to be at full strength for each dynamic effort front pause squat set.

Target Area: Dynamic Warm-Up
Band Pull-Aparts - 3 sets of 25 reps
Medicine Ball Thoracic Extension - 3 sets of 5 deep breaths
Dumbbell "T" Balance - 3 sets of 8 reps per leg

Intensity Technique: Dynamic Effort
Barbell Front Pause Squat - 4 sets of 3 reps at 55% max weight

Intensity Technique: PSD
Perform 2 sets of the following:

Set	Technique	Exercise	Reps
Set A	Pre-Exhaust	Dumbbell Lateral Raise	8–12 reps
Set B	Strength	Dumbbell Shoulder Press	6–8 reps
Set C	Drop Set	Dumbbell Lateral Raise	10+ reps

Tier 3: Posterior Chain (Upper)
Cable or Band Face Pull - 2 sets of 15 reps

Tier 3: Posterior Chain (Lower)
TRX or Physioball Single Leg Curl - 2 sets of 10 reps per leg

WEEK 7
Workout #1: Bench and Jump Power Day

WORKOUT NOTES

- Add weight to the incline bench press.
- Add weight to the dumbbell single arm snatch if you feel confident in your technique.

Target Area: Dynamic Warm-Up
Single Leg Glute Bridge (foot elevated on bench) - 3 sets of 12 reps per leg
Yoga Push-Ups - 3 sets of 10 reps
PVC Bench Thoracic Extension - 3 sets of 5 deep breaths

Intensity Technique: PAP Power
Alternate sets:
1A. Dumbbell Incline Bench Press - 3 sets of 3 reps at 70% max weight
1B. Plyo (clap) Push-Ups - 3 sets of 5 reps

Tier 1: Olympic Strength
Dumbbell Single Arm Snatch - 3 sets of 5 reps per arm

Tier 2: Carry
Dumbbell Single Arm Farmers Walks - 2 sets of 20–30 yards per side

Tier 3: Posterior Chain (Lower)
3D Barbell Hip Thrust (mini band or slingshot around the knees) - 2 sets of 15 reps

WEEK 7
Workout #2: Speed Day

WORKOUT NOTES

- See Appendix A: Speed Development Playbook on GetFitNow.com for a full dynamic warm-up.
- Added sets to the over speed drill.
- For the over speed drill, the band, bungee or tow strap should only pull/assist/force the athlete to run faster 5–10% for the first 5–10 yards or 3–5 strides. After that, release the athlete and allow them to finish the sprint.
- New change of direction drill.
- Athletes should be in small groups to race for Speed Development (Change of Direction) drills.

Target Area: Dynamic Warm-Up

Target Area: Mobility
Lunge Yoga Rotation - 2 sets of 10 reps per side
Linear Leg Swings - 2 sets of 10 reps per side
    Cue "TOES UP!"
Lateral Leg Swings - 2 sets of 10 reps per side
    Cue "TOES UP!"
Active Prehab: Ankle Mobility - 2 sets of 10 reps per side
    Hold the top of your yoga push-up position and alternate driving your knees forward to mobilize your ankles.

Tier 2: Rotation
Partner Medicine Ball Shuffle Rotation Throws - 3 sets of 5 reps per direction
    Stand as far as possible from your partner to catch the ball in the air. Take a step further away from each other each rep you catch. Take a step closer to each other if you drop the ball.

Target Area: Speed Development (Over Speed)
Light Assist (Band, Bungee, or Tow Strap) Sprint - 6 sets of 20–30 yards

Target Area: Speed Development (Acceleration)
Moderate Sled Push - 6 sets at 30–50% of your body weight

Target Area: Speed Development (Change of Direction)

Ice Skater Jumps to Forward Sprint - 4 sets of 20 yard sprints

"T" Drill - 4 sets

Set up cones in a "T" pattern, 5 yards apart. Sprint cone to cone. 5 yards forward, 5 yards lateral shuffle LEFT, 10 yards lateral shuffle RIGHT, 5 yard lateral shuffle LEFT, and 5 yards backwards to the original cone.

Cool down stretch and foam roll massage

WEEK 7
Workout #3: PAP Sled Push Day

WORKOUT NOTES

- Add weight to the sled push
- Attempt more reps in your rest/pause pull-up or chin-up sets.
- For the rest/pause set: Performing a set at 80% max effort, followed by 3–5 deep breaths, then a second max effort set, followed by 3–5 deep breaths, and finally a third max effort set, constitutes 1 "set" of rest/pause. Each round of a rest/pause set should see diminishing rep counts as you push yourself.

Target Area: Dynamic Warm-Up
PVC or Empty Barbell Overhead Squat - 3 sets of 10 reps
Walking Lunge with Rotation - 3 sets of 10 reps per leg
Band Overhead Squat Pattern - 3 sets of 10 reps

Intensity Technique: PAP Power
Alternate sets
1A. Heavy Sled Push (1.25x Body Weight) - 3 sets of 10 yards
1B. Broad Jump TRIPLES - 3 sets of 2 reps
    TRIPLES = 3 consecutive broad jumps

Intensity Technique: Rest/Pause
Pull-Up or Chin-Up - 2 sets

Tier 2: Lunge
Dumbbell Lateral Lunge - 2 sets of 12 reps per side

Tier 3: Posterior Chain (Upper)
Dumbbell Supported Row - 3 sets of 12 reps

WEEK 7
Workout #4: Speed Day

WORKOUT NOTES

- See Appendix A: Speed Development Playbook on GetFitNow.com for a full dynamic warm-up.
- Increase distance on the acceleration and sprint drills.
- Athletes should be in small groups to race for Speed Development (Change of Direction) drills.

Target Area: Dynamic Warm-Up

Target Area: Mobility
Lunge Yoga Rotation - 2 sets of 10 reps per side
Linear Leg Swings - 2 sets of 10 reps per side
    Cue "TOES UP!"
Lateral Leg Swings - 2 sets of 10 reps per side
    Cue "TOES UP!"
Active Prehab: Ankle Mobility - 2 sets of 10 reps per side
    Hold the top of your yoga push-up position and alternate driving your knees
        forward to mobilize your ankles.

Tier 2: Jump (Lateral Plyometrics)
Outside Edge (X-over) Lateral Line Bound with Stabilization - 3 sets of 8 reps per leg
    Hop off of the outside edge of your foot (X-over) from left to right/right to left
        along the lines of the track at a 45-degree angle. Stick each landing.

Target Area: Speed Development (Reaction Agility)
(Cognitive) Pro Agility (5–10–5) Drill - 6 sets
    Sprint left on "EVEN NUMBER" and sprint right on "ODD NUMBER."

Target Area: Speed Development (Acceleration)
Resisted (Band or Bungee) - 6 sets of 20 yards

Target Area: Speed Development (Sprint)
Flying 30's - 8 sets
    Build up your speed to a 30-yard full effort sprint.
Cool down stretch and foam roll massage

WEEK 7
Workout #5: Dynamic Effort Front Squat Day

WORKOUT NOTES

- Add weight to the front pause squat this week.
- Add weight to the dumbbell shoulder press in the PSD set, if possible.

Target Area: Dynamic Warm-Up
Band Pull-Aparts - 3 sets of 25 reps
Medicine Ball Thoracic Extension - 3 sets of 5 deep breaths
Dumbbell "T" Balance - 3 sets of 8 reps per leg

Intensity Technique: Dynamic Effort
Barbell Front Pause Squat - 4 sets of 3 reps at 60% max weight

Intensity Technique: PSD
Perform 2 sets of the following:

Set	Technique	Exercise	Reps
Set A	Pre-Exhaust	Dumbbell Lateral Raise	8–12 reps
Set B	Strength	Dumbbell Shoulder Press	6–8 reps
Set C	Drop Set	Dumbbell Lateral Raise	10+ reps

Tier 3: Posterior Chain (Upper)
Cable or Band Face Pull - 2 sets of 15 reps

Tier 3: Posterior Chain (Lower)
TRX or Physioball Single Leg Curl - 3 sets of 10 reps per leg

WEEK 8
Workout #1: Bench and Jump Power Day

WORKOUT NOTES

- Increase volume (reps and sets) on assistance work.

Target Area: Dynamic Warm-Up
Single Leg Glute Bridge (foot elevated on bench) - 3 sets of 12 reps per leg
Yoga Push-Ups - 3 sets of 10 reps
PVC Bench Thoracic Extension - 3 sets of 5 deep breaths

Intensity Technique: PAP Power
Alternate sets:
1A. Dumbbell Incline Bench Press - 3 sets of 3 reps at 70% max weight
1B. Plyo (clap) Push-Ups - 3 sets of 5 reps

Tier 1: Olympic Strength
Dumbbell Single Arm Snatch - 3 sets of 5 reps each arm

Tier 2: Carry
Dumbbell Single Arm Farmers Walks - 3 sets of 20–30 yards each side

Tier 3: Posterior Chain (Lower)
3D Barbell Hip Thrust (mini band or slingshot around the knees) - 4 sets of 8 reps

WEEK 8
Workout #2: Speed Day

WORKOUT NOTES

- See Appendix A: Speed Development Playbook on GetFitNow.com for a full dynamic warm-up.
- Added volume to the acceleration drill.
- For the over speed drill, the band, bungee or tow strap should only pull/assist/force the athlete to run faster 5–10% for the first 5–10 yards or 3–5 strides. After that, release it and finish the sprint normally.
- New change of direction drill.
- Athletes should be in small groups to race for Speed Development (Change of Direction) drills.

Target Area: Dynamic Warm-Up

Target Area: Mobility
Lunge Yoga Rotation - 2 sets of 10 reps per side
Linear Leg Swings - 2 sets of 10 reps per side
    Cue "TOES UP!"
Lateral Leg Swings - 2 sets of 10 reps per side
    Cue "TOES UP!"
Active Prehab: Ankle Mobility - 2 sets of 10 reps per side
    Hold the top of your yoga push-up position and alternate driving your knees forward to mobilize your ankles.

Tier 2: Rotation
Partner Medicine Ball Shuffle Rotation Throws - 3 sets of 5 reps each direction
    Stand as far as possible from your partner to catch the ball in the air. Take a step further away from each other each rep you catch. Take a step closer to each other if you drop the ball.

Target Area: Speed Development (Over Speed)
Light Assist (Band, Bungee, or Tow Strap) Sprint - 6 sets of 20–30 yards

Target Area: Speed Development (Acceleration)
Moderate Sled Push - 8 sets at 30–50% of your body weight

VARSITY LEVEL   PRE-SEASON II [WINTER]

Target Area: Speed Development (Change of Direction)
"T" Drill - 4 sets
> Set up cones in a "T" pattern, 5 yards apart. Sprint cone to cone. 5 yards
> forward, 5 yards lateral shuffle LEFT, 10 yards lateral shuffle RIGHT, 5
> yard lateral shuffle LEFT, and 5 yards backwards to the original cone.

3-Cone Drill - 4 sets
Cool down stretch and foam roll massage

WEEK 8
Workout #3: PAP Sled Push Day

WORKOUT NOTES

- Increase volume (reps and sets) on assistance work.
- For the rest/pause set: Performing a set at 80% max effort, followed by 3–5 deep breaths, then a second max effort set, followed by 3–5 deep breaths, and finally a third max effort set, constitutes 1 "set" of rest/pause. Each round of a rest/pause set should see diminishing rep counts as you push yourself.

Target Area: Dynamic Warm-Up
PVC or Empty Barbell Overhead Squat - 3 sets of 10 reps
Walking Lunge with Rotation - 3 sets of 10 reps per leg
Band Overhead Squat Pattern - 3 sets of 10 reps

Intensity Technique: PAP Power
Alternate sets:
1A. Heavy Sled Push (1.25x Body Weight) - 3 sets of 10 yards
1B. Broad Jump TRIPLES - 3 sets of 2 reps
    TRIPLES = 3 consecutive broad jumps.

Intensity Technique: Rest/Pause
Pull-Up or Chin-Up - 2 sets

Tier 2: Lunge
Dumbbell Lateral Lunge - 4 sets of 8 reps per side

Tier 3: Posterior Chain (Upper)
Dumbbell Supported Row - 3 sets of 12 reps

WEEK 8
Workout #4: Speed Day

WORKOUT NOTES

- See Appendix A: Speed Development Playbook on GetFitNow.com for a full dynamic warm-up.
- Increase difficulty on lateral plyometrics exercise by doing double jumps.
- Increase distance on sprint drill.
- Athletes should be in small groups to race for Speed Development (Change of Direction) drills.

Target Area: Dynamic Warm-Up

Target Area: Mobility
Lunge Yoga Rotation - 2 sets of 10 reps per side
Linear Leg Swings - 2 sets of 10 reps per side
    Cue "TOES UP!"
Lateral Leg Swings - 2 sets of 10 reps per side
    Cue "TOES UP!"
Active Prehab: Ankle Mobility - 2 sets of 10 reps per side
    Hold the top of your yoga push-up position and alternate driving your knees
        forward to mobilize your ankles.

Tier 2: Jump (Lateral Plyometrics)
Outside Edge (X-over) Lateral Line Bound with Stabilization - 3 sets of 8 reps per leg
    Perform two consecutive ("double") hops off the outside edge of your foot
        (X-over) from left to right/right to left along the lines of the track at a
        45-degree angle. Stick each landing.

Target Area: Reaction Agility
(Cognitive) Pro Agility (5–10–5) Drill - 6 sets
    Sprint left on "EVEN NUMBER" and sprint right on "ODD NUMBER."

Target Area: Speed Development (Acceleration)
Resisted (Band or Bungee) High Knee Sprint - 6 sets of 20 yards

Target Area: Speed Development (Sprint)
Flying 40's - 8 sets
    Build up your speed to a 40-yard full effort sprint.
Cool down stretch and foam roll massage

WEEK 8
Workout #5: Dynamic Effort Front Squat Day

WORKOUT NOTES

- Increase volume (reps and sets) on assistance work.

Target Area: Dynamic Warm-Up
Band Pull-Aparts - 3 sets of 25 reps
Medicine Ball Thoracic Extension - 3 sets of 5 deep breaths
Dumbbell "T" Balance - 3 sets of 8 reps per leg

Intensity Technique: Dynamic Effort
Barbell Front Pause Squat - 4 sets of 3 reps at 60% max weight

Intensity Technique: PSD
Perform 2 sets of the following:

Set	Technique	Exercise	Reps
Set A	Pre-Exhaust	Dumbbell Lateral Raise	8–12 reps
Set B	Strength	Dumbbell Shoulder Press	6–8 reps
Set C	Drop Set	Dumbbell Lateral Raise	10+ reps

Tier 3: Posterior Chain (Upper)
Cable or Band Face Pull - 3 sets of 20 reps

Tier 3: Posterior Chain (Lower)
TRX or Physioball Single Leg Curl - 4 sets of 10 reps per leg

PRE-SEASON II (WINTER)   VARSITY LEVEL

THE IRON FALCON PROGRAM

This program was created to generate healthy competition in the weight room, using quantifiable athletic movements that will give athletes the physical tools to become baseball players. The goals on this chart were designed for those working to become college baseball players.

PROGRAM NOTES

This program uses relative strength ratios to create gender-specific IRON FALCON programs. Please refer back to the section on Strength Ratios on page 130. All barbell exercises are based on a 5-rep max at 85–87 percent of a 1-rep max effort. I believe the 5 rep range is best for high school athletes because it improves strength and technical efficiency.

HOW TO BECOME AN IRON FALCON

Over my 15 years at The Peddie School, I have had many permutations of the IRON FALCON program. Here is my current protocol:

#1: Reach eight Iron Falcon goals of the ten Lift/Strength exercises, based on relative strength goals:

1. Barbell Front Squat
2. Barbell Back Squat
3. Barbell Deadlift
4. Barbell RDL
5. Barbell Shoulder Press
6. Trap Bar Deadlift
7. Barbell Hang Clean
8. Dumbbell Bench Press
9. Dumbbell Bulgarian Squat
10. Pull-up

VARSITY LEVEL — PRE-SEASON II (WINTER)

#2: Reach two Iron Falcon GOALS of the four Speed, Agility, and Power exercises:

1. 10 yard Sprint (Acceleration)
   a. Boys = 1.6 seconds
   b. Girls = 1.75 seconds

2. 10 yard Flying Sprint
   a. Boys = 19.5 mph
   b. Girls = 17.5 mph

3. Vertical Jump
   a. Boys = 30 inches
   b. Girls = 24 inches

4. Pro Agility 5-10-5
   a. Boys = 4.35 seconds
   b. Girls = 4.7 seconds

Bonus points are available for those who demonstrate the particular character traits I aim to build in my high school athletes. Juniors and Seniors can earn a maximum of two of the following bonuses:

- **Consistency:** Attended every workout

- **Scholarship:** Grade Point Average

- **Discipline:** Two Varsity Sport Athlete

A final note on the IRON FALCON program: Ultimately, *you* have to pick exercises, target weights and times for those exercises that are best for your team, your program, and your facility.

THE HIGH SCHOOL ATHLETE HOT TOPIC SERIES: MEDICINE BALL TENNIS

This is easily the most fun game you have never played! A well-played game of medicine ball tennis between a couple varsity baseball players pays so many physical and emotional dividends: it creates rotational power every time you throw the ball; trains deceleration and grip strength every time you catch the ball; improves acceleration and instincts every time you chase the ball; builds communication and teamwork between the players; encourages competition…and above all else, it's fun!

Essentially, this game is 2 on 2 tennis with a medicine ball, but there are a few specific rules to go over. Check us out on Instagram @VolkmarPerformance for some example videos of kids playing.

THE BASICS

The game is played with two players per team. Freshman and JV players can use 4 lbs., 6 lbs., or 8 lbs. medicine balls; varsity players can use 10 or 12 lbs. balls. The game is designed to be played on an outside tennis court with doubles lines, but an indoor court can be made with cones outlining the court and folding chairs as the net.

Players *must* alternate shots, as this creates more movement and teamwork. We play games to 5 points to rotate more players in, but you can play games to 3 points or 11 points, depending on the goal of the exercise. First team to the designated score wins!

THE SERVE

The serve is done from behind the doubles end line (if outside) or the cones end line (if inside). The goal of the serve is to throw the ball as high and far as possible, pushing your opponent as far back as possible to their own end line. You may give players one or two shuffle steps to create more momentum to create longer serves if needed. Each player alternates the serve.

RECEIVING AND RETURNING THE SERVE

Either player may receive the serve, which may be caught while the ball is in the air or on the bounce, but if dropped, the point is awarded to the other team. If the serve gets past both athletes, or bounces twice, it is considered an ACE, and the point is awarded to the other team.

THE VOLLEY

This is the most important rule of the game: The athlete who did not serve returns the volley. Similarly, on the other team, the athlete who did not *receive* the serve returns the volley. Simply put, all players must *alternate* shots throughout play. Both sides continue to alternate catching the volley until the point is over. A point is scored when the ball is dropped, thrown out of bounds, touches the net, or bounces twice.

You get one step, a pivot foot (like basketball) and a shuffle step to catch and throw the ball. You cannot pause before you return the throw, and must volley the ball back as quickly as possible. It is up to the net judge to call shot clock violations if an athlete takes too long to return a shot.

The medicine ball can be thrown in any manner—*except* like a baseball. This puts too much stress on the elbow and shoulder.

You may save the ball from going out of bounds, but if an athlete is heading out of bounds, they must catch the ball *in* bounds and pass it to a teammate before landing out of bounds.

VARIATIONS
3-on-3 Zone Defense

I typically do this variation with younger, weaker players, as 3 on 3 gets more players involved in a single game. All other rules apply, except now any kid can make a play on the ball. This allows for younger players to make longer volleys and calls for more teamwork because now the players have to communicate better as to who is going to field each ball.

THE HIGH SCHOOL ATHLETE HOT TOPIC SERIES: BOX SQUATS 101

I love the box squat. You see it in my Progression/Advancement of Core Lifts table on pages 65–66; as part of my Building to the Barbell Front Squat progression on page 74; and it features prominently in the off-season and the pre-season programs in this book.

The box squat is incredibly versatile, with both athletes and coaches able to adjust it to suit their goals and abilities. For that reason, I wanted to go into a bit more detail on how best to perform, as well as modify, the box squat.

HEIGHT

Broadly speaking, the box squat can be performed from three different height categories:

1. **High box (above parallel).** This overloads the squat to produce greater vertical force. Athletes at the NBA Combine don't perform a full squat before they jump, you'll notice—they do a super-fast ¼-squat with rapid arm movement. A higher box can also help a younger, taller athlete new to the barbell squat.

2. **Parallel box.** Maintaining proper squat depth, this is the standard for box squats.

3. **Low (below parallel).** A lower height emphasizes mobility during the GPP phase.

Choosing the ideal box height (typically between 12–18 inches) will be dependent on your ability to maintain a neutral spinal and pelvic position while in contact with the box. It is **very important** that you position the box only as low as you can maintain a neutral spine and core stability! Athletes of the same height may still need different box heights based on their anatomy. When in doubt, position the box higher and earn the right to lower it over time.

ADVANTAGES OF THE BOX SQUAT

- **Produces greater acceleration strength.** Overcoming a pause at the bottom forces the athlete to produce more force to Squat up.

- **Can be programmed to be height-specific.**

- **Builds confidence in younger lifters.**

- **Re-teaches proper depth efficiently for new athletes.** Every program gets at least one new athlete who claims the ability to do a "3 plate squat," but does it with ½ or ¼ depth. A 14–16-inch box does not lie.

- **Builds core stability at the bottom of the squat.** Athletes tend to relax their lower back and rock back on the box. Some even allow the lumbar spine to flex. This is a *huge* injury risk. Maintaining core stability and a neutral spine needs to be constantly reinforced and monitored.

- **Gives better ability to teach the hinge technique.** Younger athletes can confidently hinge backwards knowing they have a box to aim for/sit on.

- **Builds more posterior chain (glutes, hamstrings, and low back) strength.** A slightly wider stance and more hinge at the hips (driving your hips back first before the knees bend) means more glutes, hamstrings, adductors, and low back muscle activation.

- **The perfect mid- to late-season exercise.** Creating less soreness than the traditional Squat, less stress on the knees (with the greater emphasis on pushing the hips back) and offering the chance to unload the spine and low back with a high box…it's no wonder I love the box squat!

ACKNOWLEDGMENTS

To my family: my loving wife Kelly, to MJ and Tay Tay. Thank all of you so much. You had so much patience while I was pursuing this project. Tay Tay especially, you watched endless movies while I was in the office. I love you princess.

To all the baseball athletes at all levels I have coached: Thank you for your hard work and dedication to the program.

To my Peddie School baseball coach, Coach Eric Treese: You trusted me with the future of your program, and for that, I thank you.

To the Peddie School: You have allowed me to practice and hone my craft for the last 15 years. Thank you for that opportunity.

To Bruce Peditto: You were a neighborhood friend, who turned into an intern, who turned into a colleague, who turned into a strength coach in professional baseball, but most important, you turned into a friend who helped edit this book.

To Jon and Greg Schwind: You both put me in touch with the man whose name is on the cover of this book. That door would not have opened without either of you. Also, thank you for your stories and edits for this book.

To Andrew, Ryan T, and Ryan K: You continue to take a strength coach's word and ideas and design them into an easy-to-understand resource for all.

All of you are an inspiration in my life, and it is through my life experiences that my books are shaped.

FIND MORE *HIGH SCHOOL ATHLETE* TIPS ON GETFITNOW!

Visit GetFitNow.com to download additional program resources, including a detailed exercise database and point-by-point playbooks covering speed development, improving vertical jumps, and much more.

EVIDENCE-BASED

SCAN: Sports, Cardiovascular, and Wellness Nutrition Group
scandpg.org
SCAN is a dietetic practice group of the Academy of Nutrition and Dietetics

NCAA Sports Science Institute
ncaa.org/health-and-safety/sport-science-institute
The NCAA Sport Science Institute (SSI) is a new national center for the study and improvement of health and safety in athletics

Precision Nutrition
precisionnutrition.com
Precision Nutrition is the home of the world's top nutrition coaches, offering many free articles and tips. They have worked with many professional organizations and athletes.

My Sports Dietitian
mysportsd.com
This website offers multiple free resources and apps that can help all athletes.

The National Strength and Conditioning Association
nsca.com
The NSCA offers an abundance of sports nutrition information and research to its members and coaches.

International Society of Sports Nutrition
sportsnutritionsociety.org
The International Society of Sports Nutrition is the only non-profit academic society dedicated to promoting the science and application of evidence-based sports nutrition and supplementation.

5/3/1 Program
jimwendler.com

The Ultimate Pull-Up Program
Meghan Callaway

Recovery Strategies
Powerful Recovery Methods by Joe Hashey

AthletesAcceleration.com
athletesacceleration.com

Complete Guide to Training the Female Athlete by Adam Feit and Bobby Smith

Complete Jumps Training: The Coaches Guide to Jump Training by Adam Feit and Bobby Smith

Rutgers Football Performance Nutrition Manual
Dylan Klein, PhD, Assistant Professor, Health & Exercise Science, Rowan University
Please contact Dylan for nutrition consults at decline104@gmail.com.

Lafayette College
Sports Nutrition Handbook

Conscious Coaching: The Art and Science of Building Buy-In
Brett Bartholomew

Movement Over Maxes
Zach Dechant

Adam Feit, MS, CSCS*D, RSCC, SCCC, PN2
Coordinator of Physical and Mental Performance
Doctoral Candidate: Sport and Exercise Psychology
afeit@springfield.edu
@strengthpsych
@strengthpsychcoach

Midwest Orthopedics at Rush in Chicago, Illinois
rushortho.com

Conscious Coaching: The Art and Science of Building Buy-In
Brett Bartholomew

Triphasic Training
Cal Dietz and Ben Peterson

Movement Over Maxes
Zach Dechant

Journal of Athletic Training
natajournals.org

National Strength and Conditioning Association (NSCA)
Provides the ten pillars for successful long-term athletic development.

usabltad.com
The Long-Term Athlete Development (LTAD) Model developed by MLB
and USA Baseball

FITNESS TRACKING

TeamBuildr
TeamBuildr is a strength and conditioning software platform that allows coaches to build workouts online, distribute workouts paperless, and collect data for tracking and reporting purposes. It includes an exercise library that comes with preloaded exercises, videos and training programs, along with a full training template library, which includes sport-specific and performance-specific programming.

NUTRITION TRACKING

I suggest following a few college sports nutrition program on social media:

- @calsportsnutrition
- @fuelingbruins
- @dukesportsnutrition

Eat 2 Win Nutrition

- Track and log their eating habits with guidance from unique and customized meal plans
- Create a team challenge and encourage group competition and engagement
- Athletes can choose to give permission to certain key people to view, comment and rate their eating habits based on the pictures of the food they are eating.

MyFitnessPal

- One of the most popular, comprehensive nutrition and fitness apps
- Offers a set of features to track fitness as well as tracking food
- By far the most integrations with wearable fitness devices

Fooducate

- A free app that grades your player's food using a unique grading system
- Each food item in their database comes with a letter grade (A, B, C, etc.) so it's easy for the user to evaluate the quality of that food item
- Gives the players an opportunity to learn quality food choices

ABOUT THE AUTHOR

Michael Volkmar, MS, CSCS, PES, CPT, received his master's degree in Exercise Science with a specialization in Exercise, Nutrition, and Eating Behavior from George Washington University (GWU). He worked for three years as the Strength and Conditioning Coach at GWU before moving on to spend one year at the International Performance Institute of IMG Academies, FL. Mike continued his professional development by becoming the Director of Strength and Conditioning at the APEX Academies. Currently, Mike is in his 16th season as the strength and conditioning coach at the Peddie School. He has advanced specialty certifications in strength and conditioning, post-rehab exercise, athletic development, and sports medicine.

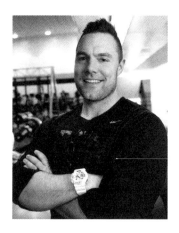

ALSO AVAILABLE

The Dumbbell Workout Handbook: Strength and Power
The Dumbbell Workout Handbook: Weight Loss
Gymnastic Rings Workout Handbook
The High School Athlete: Basketball
The High School Athlete: Football
The Mobility Workout Handbook
Strong Legs
Tabata Workout Handbook, Volume 2